DUTCH OVEN COOKBOOK 2021

RECIPES TO ENJOY WITH YOUR WHOLE FAMILY

Table of Contents

Rice pudding

Marzipan wreath with pumpkin

Potato pancakes

Crumble with blueberries

Tarte

Bread with fruits

Waffles

Sweet potato bread

Bread with olives

Hefezopf

Omelette with mushrooms

Pull apart bread

Walnut bread with apple

Main courses

Rolled roast with mozzarella and mushrooms

Chili con carne

Wild walnut salmon

Stuffed bread

Vegetable quiche

Lasagna with spinach

Pumpkin curry

Squid stew

Cinnamon ribs on orange

Bean stew

Pizza mozzarella

Layer meat

Stew pot with onions

Beef with pineapple curry

Potatoes with meat in the pot

Creole Jambalaya

Cauliflower risotto with minced meat

Cheese noodles

Rice with vegetables and banana

Coq au vin

Hack in the cabbage coat

Curry with tofu

Sweet and sour duck

Bolognese

Macaroni cheese

Crispy redfish

Sharp ribs

Stuffed peppers

Mince casserole with mushrooms

Chicken leg on beans

Moussaka

Lamb shank

Sweet Potato Curry

Risotto with asparagus

Pulled Pork

Pumpkin with mince

Shrimp with coconut

Stew with zucchini

Noodle pot

Mediterranean brisket

Soups

Chicken Cheese Soup

Chestnut Pumpkin Soup

Chorizo potato soup

Lentil soup

Cheese and potato soup

Tomato soup

Zucchini soup

Chicken soup

Rice and lemon soup

Avocado with potato soup

Peppery soup

Sauerkraut soup

Wild West soup

Spinach in wild garlic soup

Apple soup with red cabbage

Snacks

Cinnamon rolls

Nutcake

Caramelized almonds

Elderberry dumplings

Popcorn

Cheese   pretzels

Covered Maultaschen

Raspberry cream in puff pastry

Apple rings

Two kinds of Americans

Halloumnis skewers

Onion rings in buttermilk

Fish Patties

Ratatouille

Filled mushrooms

Bread with garlic butter

Oat patty

Potato gratin

Vegetables with feta

Preface

Dutch Oven ... what is that? Many camping and outdoor fans are gradually becoming aware of the Dutch Oven. The trend is slowly spilling over from the USA to us in Germany and more and more people are enthusiastic about this all-rounder. This cast iron pot is a real all-rounder and perfect for cooking in the wilderness, camping or at home over the fireplace.

Whether soups, stews, steaks, cakes, bread or fried eggs, with the Dutch Oven you can cook pretty much anything in the great outdoors. In this book you will find our 111 best Dutch Oven recipes sorted by breakfast, main dishes, soups, snacks, side dishes and pastries & desserts. You will also find an introduction to cooking with the Dutch Oven, the interesting story behind it, how to best use it and what to look out for when cooking. There is also nutritional information on all 111 recipes. No matter whether you are a beginner or a professional, this book is suitable for everyone and offers both classics and varied and interesting recipes.

Have fun cooking with the Dutch Oven!

Food revolution

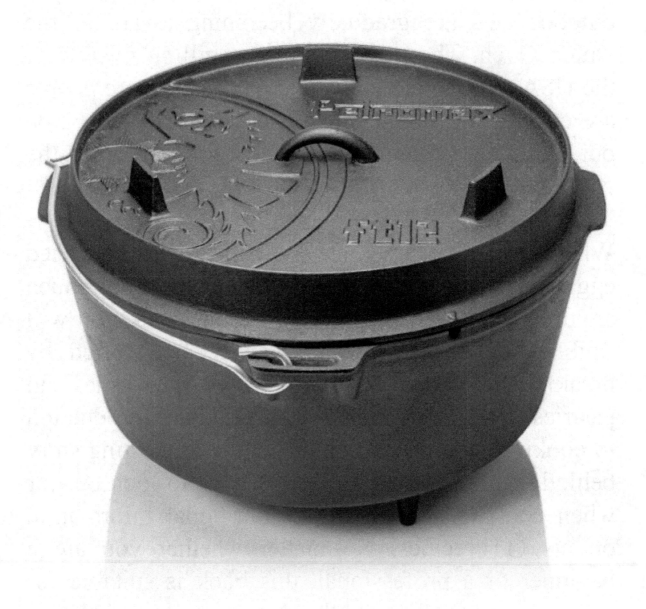

Dutch Oven - everything you need to know

What is a Dutch Oven?

One hears and reads more and more frequently about a "Dutch Oven". Your Dutch Oven, also known as DO or Dopf, is a pot made of solid cast iron. Dutch ovens have been around for over 300 years and they are still used by many people for cooking. A DO has thick walls made of cast iron and a tightly fitting lid. The lid can be covered with coal or briquettes and heated with it. The lid has a high edge so that the coal or ashes do not fall into the food when the lid is lifted.

In addition, depending on the variant, the Dutch Oven has three legs so that it can be placed safely over hot coals. Many models also have a handle so that the pot can be hung over a campfire. The thick cast iron stores heat very well and, above all, for a long time, and because it is heated from above and below, a Dutch oven can be compared to a mobile oven. The heat is distributed very well and, depending on the dish, the top / bottom heat can be individually adjusted or set.

These properties made the Dutch Oven popular with American pioneers back then. Even today it is the absolute favorite with campers and fans of the outdoor kitchen when it comes to cooking. In South Africa it is called Potje, in the USA and Australia Dopf or Camp Oven. When used correctly, a Dutch Oven is very robust and will last for many years.

The Dopf is available as an outdoor version and as an indoor version without legs and handles. So it can be used on the stove or in the oven.

A Dutch Oven is very versatile and, when closed, is like a mobile oven. Everything that can be prepared in the oven can also be prepared in the pot. Whether bread, meat, pastries, roasts or cakes - with the Dutch Oven this is no problem. Soups and stews can also be used as a pot and the lid can be used as a pan for frying or as a baking tray. In this way, numerous delicious dishes can be conjured up in the great outdoors.

In summary, a Dutch Oven is an oven, pot, pan and baking tray in one.

The size is given in quart (QT for short = 0.95 liters) or in inches (i.e. diameter). The important thing is how many liters fit in the DO. Depending on the purpose or for how many people you want to use your Dutch Oven, it should be neither too big nor too small.

The following breakdown can serve as a rough guide:
1l - 2l: for sauces and desserts
2l - 3l: for 1 - 3 people
4l - 5l: for 2 - 5 people
6l - 8l: for 4 - 8 people
8l - 10l: for 8 - 14 people

You should also keep in mind that the pots are not dishwasher safe and must be hand washed - depending on the size of your sink, this can be tricky.

The history of the Dutch Oven is not clear and there are various theories. The most common is that of the Englishman Abraham Darby. The Dutch were way ahead of the English in cast iron production and so in 1704 Abraham Darby decided to travel to Holland and learn cast iron production from the Dutch there. A few years later Darby traveled back to England and patented a similar production process for cast iron there. Since it was very similar to those used by the Dutch, it was called the Dutch Oven. The Dutch Oven has been around for over 300 years.

In the 19th century, the Dutch Oven began to conquer the United States. During the colonization of the western United States, many settlers and pioneers used the Dutch Oven. With it they could cook over open fires or coals anywhere in the wilderness and prepare so many delicious dishes. The Dutch Oven was so valuable to the settlers that it was inherited and in some cases passed on from generation to generation. The stew is still very popular in the USA and, for example, the official state cooking pot in Texas. The trend is gradually spilling over to us in Germany and more and more people are using a

Dutch oven for cooking at home or in the great outdoors.

Before a new Dutch Oven can be used, it should first be burned in. Because new pots are coated with a protective layer of wax and can have residues and soiling from production.

The patina is created during baking. This is a non-stick coating (similar to Teflon) and protects the Dutch Oven from corrosion. First clean the pot thoroughly from the inside with lukewarm water and a little washing-up liquid. This should be the first and last time your Dutch Oven comes into contact with dish soap. There are surfactants in detergents - these dissolve grease and thus destroy the patina.

After you have cleaned your Dutch Oven, you should dry it thoroughly or wipe it dry. Then rub your DO inside and out with oil (e.g. coconut oil). Then you place it with the opening facing down on a grillage and burn it at about 250 ° C for about 1.5 hours. Alternatively, a gas grill can be used for this. The third option is to put the pot upside down in the oven (place aluminum foil under the pot) and burn it for about 1.5 hours at 250 ° C. When burning in the oven, some of the oil evaporates and a lot of smoke can develop - therefore ventilate the kitchen well!

The pores of the cast iron open up due to the heat, so that the oil can penetrate them and the protective layer is created. This black layer is the patina. The more you use your stew, the darker and "better" the patina becomes. Since the patina is still quite "weak" after baking, you should not prepare any acidic dishes at the beginning.

After baking, wipe it with a dry cloth and that's it. Some manufacturers do the initial branding for you - pay attention to this when buying.

In principle, a Dutch Oven is very easy to care for. After each use, remove all leftover food and rinse thoroughly with lukewarm water. It is best to remove burnt-in residues with a wooden spade. After cleaning, dry thoroughly and coat the inside with a thin layer of oil.

NEVER use dish soap or put the Dutch Oven in the dishwasher. Detergent and soap destroy the patina and the saucepan absorbs the detergent - the next time you use it, your food will have a soapy aftertaste.

Brand new

It can happen that the Dutch Oven has to be re-baked because the patina has been destroyed / damaged, it has gone rancid or has started to rust. Then simply clean with a steel sponge and lukewarm water until the black patina has been removed. Brand new and the Dutch Oven can be used again.

You should follow a few important tips for storing and handling your Dutch Oven - so you can use it for a long time and don't have to re-brand it. A pot should always be stored dry and the lid must never close the pot tightly. Otherwise the oil inside will go rancid and the food will also go rancid during preparation - you will have to re-brand your pot. Therefore, always leave a small gap so that the air can circulate inside. It is best to put a few sheets of kitchen paper inside.

The cast iron will rust quickly if you leave your pot in the water or if you don't dry it off properly on the inside. In addition, you should never leave your pot empty over a campfire or over the embers, as this can deform the cast iron and in the worst case even break.

Therefore, never put cold liquids in a hot pot. Due to the large temperature difference, the cast iron can break here too. It is also important to never leave liquids or food scraps in the DO. This can damage the patina and begin to rust. So clean quickly after use.

If you pay attention to all of this, you will enjoy your pot for a long time.

A Dutch Oven can actually be fired with pretty much any heat source. Whether campfire, open fire, gas grill, oven, charcoal or briquettes - the main thing is that enough heat is given off.

For a Dutch oven, however, it is advisable to use briquettes as they offer numerous advantages. Briquettes burn much longer than normal charcoal and are easier to dose or place at the desired location. In addition, briquettes give off heat evenly and for a very long time. Using briquettes also creates less ash. It is extremely important to be careful about choosing the right briquettes. Cheap briquettes crumble faster and burn up faster too. It is therefore not advisable to save on the briquettes.

Briquettes made from coconut are very suitable for use in a Dutch oven. These glow long and evenly and are both odorless and almost smoke-free. Coconut briquettes also don't crumble after a few hours - so there is hardly any dust and ash. Coconut briquettes are a little more expensive than normal briquettes, but they offer many advantages and are particularly suitable for long stews or stews.

The temperature depends on many factors such as wind strength, ambient temperature, air humidity, coal / briquettes used, etc. The following guidelines will help you to reach a temperature of approx. 170 ° C in the Dutch Oven:

Dutch Oven size in inches * 2
Example: 12 "* 2 = approx. 24 briquettes necessary to reach approx. 170 ° C.

Or volume of the pot * 4
Example: 6 l * 4 = approx. 24 briquettes necessary to reach approx. 170 ° C.

For pots with a size **of less than 10 "** , the following can be used as a guide for higher temperatures:

For every further 15 ° C increase in temperature (starting from 170 ° C) simply use one more briquette.
Example: 10 "DO and 215 ° C = 20 briquettes + 3 briquettes = approx. 23 briquettes necessary for 215 ° C

For pots larger **than 10 "** , the following can be used as a guide for higher temperatures:

For every further 15 ° C increase in temperature (starting from 170 ° C) simply use two more briquettes.
Example: 14 "DO and 215 ° C = 24 briquettes + 6 briquettes = approx. 30 briquettes necessary for 215 ° C

The distribution of the briquettes also plays an important role. Depending on the dish, these must be distributed differently. For dishes that are to be fried or braised, half of the briquettes are placed under the pot and half on the lid.

When bread or cakes are to be baked, ¾ of the briquettes are placed on the lid and ¼ under the pot, as top heat is required here and the dishes can burn if the bottom heat is too high.

Stews and soups need a lot of bottom heat so that they can simmer to themselves. Therefore 2/3 of the briquettes under the pot and 1/3 on the lid.

Despite these guidelines, there may be differences between dishes in the same category. That's why we've added the exact distribution to each recipe. It takes a little practice and experience to properly heat the Dutch Oven. The solid cast iron slowly absorbs heat and stores it for a very long time. It takes some time for it to "pick up speed" and to be properly heated. Many beginners use too many briquettes in the beginning and the food burns as a result - so feel better than using too much heat directly.

Tips

Here are a few tips that will make using your Dutch Ovens easier. The lid can be used very well for frying. To do this, simply turn the lid over and heat it properly from below with briquettes. This allows you to sear meat before it ends up in the stew, for example, or you can fry a steak or a fried egg in the morning. Some Dutch ovens have three small legs on the lid, alternatively a pan servant can be used.

The lid should be rotated 90 degrees regularly. If there are a lot of briquettes on the lid, hotspots can occur, which should be avoided for even cooking. If there are many briquettes under the pot, the whole pot should be rotated 90 degrees regularly.

It should be checked regularly in the pot to see whether there is still enough liquid. Otherwise it may stick or burn. If there is a lot of steam coming towards you when you lift the lid, then the pot is probably too hot. Check the fluid level regularly and add fluid if necessary.

There are accessories that make your life easier. Of course you can also do without it. A wooden box or a carrying bag is suitable for storage and transport. In this way, the Dutch Oven can be safely transported and stored from A to B.

With a pan servant, the lid quickly becomes a frying pan. A pan servant takes up hardly any space, ensures that the lid can be put down safely and ensures the necessary distance between coal / briquettes / fire and lid.

A lid lifter is always advisable. This allows the lid to be lifted safely without tipping over and the briquettes falling off. The bigger the pot, the heavier the lid - a lid lifter makes it much easier to lift and the lid stays horizontal thanks to the cross brace.

The briquettes can be safely placed in the right place with charcoal tongs without burning your hands. This should definitely be made of stainless steel - barbecue tongs made of wood or plastic are unsuitable.

A chimney starter saves a lot of time, as it allows the briquettes to be lit quickly and easily and they glow even faster.

Heat-resistant gloves are also recommended. The pot gets very hot quickly and you cannot avoid using heat-resistant gloves to handle it safely.

All of these accessories are optional but recommended. However, 300 years ago the settlers in the USA had hardly any accessories and it worked without any problems!

Notes on the recipes

Before continuing with the 111 Dutch Oven recipes, a few more pointers.

Before there is criticism because there are no pictures of the individual recipes, a brief explanation of why this is so. You really only know cookbooks with beautiful pictures and photos. These cost money, take up a lot of space and thus drive up printing costs - and thus also the price. Many cookbooks cost 20 € and more due to the many pictures and are usually too beautiful and a shame to use in the dirty kitchen or outdoors. They are often thick, unwieldy and heavy - especially in the outdoor area, everything should be as compact and handy as possible.

The finished dishes rarely look like the pictures and in our opinion rarely offer added value when cooking. The pictures are of little or no help when cooking - you can save yourself then. This cookbook does not have any pictures, this allows a price of less than 10 € and a handy pocket book format, which is ideal for the outdoor kitchen. Accordingly, it is not a shame if it gets dirty or if grease and water splashes find their way onto the book.

Each recipe is described in detail and it is very easy to cook at home. The recipes are clearly structured and are always on one page, so you don't have to scroll back and forth unnecessarily.

Cooking with the Dutch Oven is not as precise as you know it from cooking in the kitchen. It starts with the temperature and ends with the Dutch Oven itself. The temperature cannot be precisely set and depends on many different factors (weather / temperature / humidity / wind force / Dutch oven model / briquettes / etc.). So it cannot be set exactly 180 ° C or 225 ° C - which is not bad either. We always cook at around 170 ° C and, if necessary, regulate the temperature individually with more / less briquettes. That is why we do not specify the exact temperature for the individual recipes and only write down how the briquettes should be distributed. We assume a temperature of around 170 ° C for all recipes.

The same applies to the cooking times. With the Dutch Oven, the cooking time cannot be set down to the minute. It depends on the temperature and thus on many different factors. So it can be that a dish is ready 10 minutes earlier or 20 minutes later. That is why we give the cooking time in an approximate time span.

When cooking with the Dutch Oven, it depends on experience and your own gut feeling. So just try out many different recipes and feel your way step by step!

Nutritional information may vary

The nutritional information of the individual recipes can vary as different products from different manufacturers have different nutritional information. Therefore, the nutritional information serves as a rough guide.

Recipes

Breakfast

Scrambled eggs with a difference

KH 2g | EW 20g | F 30g

══

Preparation time: 20 min
Servings: 8
Difficulty: easy

ingredients
-> Coal distribution: 1/3 underneath, 2/3 on the lid

- 20 slices of bacon
- ½ bunch of parsley
- 1 ostrich egg
- salt and pepper

preparation

1.) Important: For this recipe we are not using the Dutch Oven itself, but only the lid of the Dutch Oven. The ostrich egg must first be opened carefully so that the contents can be poured into a bowl. More unusual methods may be available for this and you have to reach for the toolbox. Depending on what is easiest to do that.

2.) Use a mixer to whisk the contents of the egg. Now fry the bacon strips in the pan until crispy. Share if necessary. When all the bacon is ready, take it out of the pan and let it degrease a little on a paper towel. Now put the whisked egg in the pan and let it cook through, removing it from the bottom with a spatula as you would with a classic scrambled egg.

3.) After the whole egg is completely cooked, put the bacon back in the pan.

4.) Wash the parsley thoroughly and chop it into small pieces. Spread over the scrambled eggs and enjoy. You can of course replace the recipe with chicken eggs depending on how you prefer.

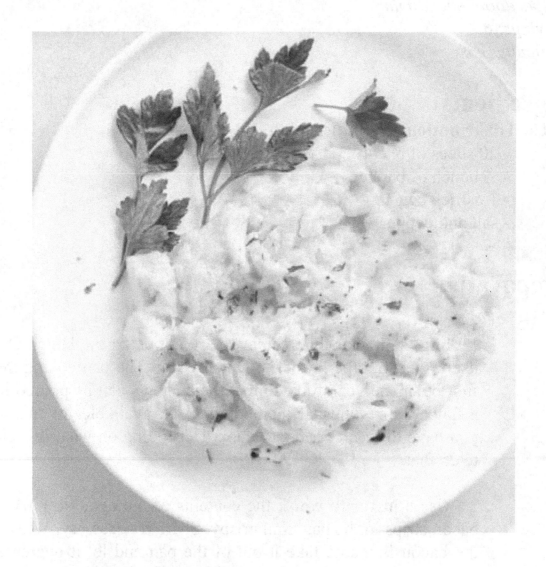

KH 85g | EW 16g | F 21g

Preparation time: 130 min + 45 min baking time
Servings: 8
Difficulty: easy

ingredients

-> **Coal distribution: ½ under the pot, ½ on the lid**

- 700g flour
- 350ml milk
- 80g sugar
- 100g butter
- 250ml cream
- 300g jam of your choice
- 9g fresh yeast
- 2 eggs
- salt

preparation

1.) Slightly warm the milk in a saucepan. Then knead into a dough with the sugar, yeast and eggs in a bowl. Then cover and let rise in a warm place.

2.) After the dough has risen, flour the work surface a little and then roll out the dough. Using a glass, cut out round, even circles. Put a teaspoon of the selected jam in the middle of each circle and seal.

3.) Pour the cream into the Dutch Oven and then spread the balls on it. In the end, this creates a kind of wreath, which can be easily divided into individual rolls. Now close the lid and let it bake for about 45 minutes.

KH 43g | EW 9g | F 3g

Preparation time: 110 min + 45 min baking time
Servings: 8
Difficulty: easy

ingredients

-> Coal distribution: 1/3 underneath, 2/3 on the lid

- 350g wheat flour
- 250ml kefir
- 200g rye flour
- 200ml of water
- 1 packet of dry yeast
- salt

preparation

1.) Put the wheat flour and the rye flour in a bowl. Add the kefir and mix everything thoroughly. Mix in the dry yeast and fill everything up with water. Knead the mixture until you get a smooth dough.

2.) Cover the bowl in a warmer place and let the dough soak for about an hour. If necessary, stretch, knead and fold a little in between.

3.) After the hour let rise, form a loaf of bread from the dough, dust with flour and let rise. Place in the Dutch Oven and cut into the top. Now bake for 45 minutes, but reduce the heat after 15 minutes.

KH 76g | EW 17g | F 11g

═══════════════════════════════════

Preparation time: 330 min + 30 min baking time
Servings: 8
Difficulty: easy

ingredients

-> Coal distribution: 1/3 underneath, 2/3 on the lid

- 1kg of flour
- 500ml milk
- 100ml of water
- 60g butter
- 20g of sugar
- 20g salt
- 20g cornstarch
- 1/2 cube of yeast

preparation

1.) Mix the water with the yeast in a bowl and add the salt. Mix everything together thoroughly and then let stand for about 3 hours in a warmer place so that the yeast can rise.

2.) Let the butter melt and add to the previous dough together with the cornstarch, milk and sugar and knead everything together. Then let it rest airtight for 2 hours. Knead again after 2 hours of rest.

3.) Place the dough on baking paper in the Dutch Oven and let it soak for the third time. After 30 minutes, bake for about half an hour.

KH 64g | EW 10g | F 14g

Preparation time: 45 min
Servings: 4
Difficulty: easy

ingredients

-> Coal distribution: 2/3 below, 1/3 on the lid

- 400ml of water
- 200ml quinoa
- 200g of different berries
- 60g walnuts (chopped)
- 4 pears
- 2 tbsp maple syrup
- 1 teaspoon of cinnamon

preparation

1.) Put the water in the Dutch Oven. Thoroughly wash the quinoa in a sieve and also put it in the Dutch Oven. Bring the water to the boil and let the quinoa soak for about 25 minutes at a lower temperature.

2.) Wash the pears thoroughly with hot water and remove the skin if you like, but important nutrients are also lost. Remove the stalk and the kernels and then dice into bite-sized pieces.

3.) Wash the berries with warm water, remove any greens and cut all fruits bite-sized. Set the berries and pear aside.

4.) As soon as the quinoa has swelled enough, divide it up, garnish with the fruit and garnish with the cinnamon, maple syrup and walnuts.

KH 35g | EW 8g | F 3g

Preparation time: 30 min
Servings: 4
Difficulty: easy

ingredients

-> Coal distribution: all briquettes under the furnace

- 175ml oat milk
- 100g oatmeal
- 100g whole wheat flour
- 50ml seltzer
- 2 ½ tbsp soy flour
- Oil of your choice for frying

preparation

1.) Only the lid of the Dutch oven is required for this recipe. Mix the soy flour with the whole wheat flour in a bowl. Add the oat milk and mix everything together thoroughly.

2.) Finally add the oat flakes and the seltzer and mix everything to a smooth batter. Let rise for 15 minutes.

3.) Preheat the lid and add the selected oil. Now use a ladle to bake the pancakes in portions and turn once as soon as the dough can no longer drip on top. Then garnish with a topping of your choice and enjoy.

KH 65g | EW 11g | F 2g

═══════════════════════════════════

Preparation time: 20 min + 60 min baking time
Servings: 8
Difficulty: easy

ingredients

-> Coal distribution: 1/3 underneath, 2/3 on the lid

- 150g whole wheat flour
- 600g flour (type 550)
- 1 ½ packets of dry yeast
- 500ml lukewarm water
- 2 tablespoons of salt and sugar
- 2 teaspoons of oil
- 15g farmer's bread spice or other spices as desired

preparation

1.) Thoroughly mix the two types of flour, the dry yeast and the lukewarm water in a bowl. Then season with the sugar and salt and round off with the farmer's bread spices.

2.) Add the oil and line the Dutch Oven with baking paper. If necessary, brush with a little oil. Pour in the dough and let it bake for about 1 hour with the lid closed.

3.) After the hour of baking time, first check whether the bread is through. Then let the dough rest for another 10 minutes.

4.) If desired, the bread can be refined with your own spices before or during the baking process. While baking is not advisable, however, as otherwise the roasted aromas cannot fully develop.

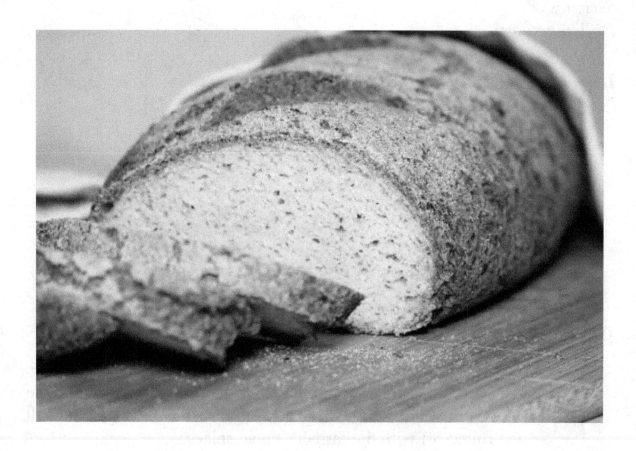

KH 30g | EW 15g | F 15g

===============

Preparation time: 45 min
Servings: 4
Difficulty: easy

ingredients

-> Coal distribution: all briquettes below

- 1.5 liters of milk
- 275g rice pudding
- 30g sugar
- some oil

preparation

1.) Heat the Dutch Oven and pour in the oil so that the whole base is covered. Also add the milk and milreis. As soon as the two components simmer for a few minutes, add the sugar and mix in.

2.) Then stir every 5 minutes until the whole rice pudding is ready after 30 minutes. Then the rice pudding can be enjoyed in portions and refined with fruits, chocolate, cinnamon, superfoods and everything your heart desires.

Marzipan wreath with pumpkin

KH 83g | EW 18g | F 32g

Preparation time: 90 min + 40 min baking time
Servings: 10
Difficulty: medium

ingredients

-> Coal distribution: 1/3 underneath, 2/3 on the lid

- 650g flour (type 630)
- 750g butternut squash
- 240ml milk
- 380g marzipan
- 200g almond leaves
- 110g butter
- 60g brown sugar
- 20g fresh yeast
- 1 egg
- 3 tbsp cinnamon
- some salt

preparation

1.) Mix the fresh yeast with the lukewarm water and 2 tablespoons of sugar in a bowl and let it swell for 10 minutes. Warm up the milk and dissolve both the butter and 180g marzipan in it. Add to the yeast mixture, mix both together.

2.) Mix both with the spelled flour and knead everything until a uniform yeast dough is formed. Cover and let the bowl soak in a warm place for 60 minutes.

3.) Peel the pumpkin and remove the seeds. Then cut into even thin slices. Divide the dough into two identical pieces and roll out thinly. For the topping, distribute the pumpkin slices and the remaining marzipan over the two pieces of dough. Now pour the almond pieces over it and sprinkle with a little sugar.

4.) Roll up the dough and then cut it into pieces about 5 cm thick. Place on baking paper in the Dutch Oven. Close the lid and bake for 40 minutes.

KH 75g | EW 13g | F 6g

Preparation time: 40 min
Servings: 8
Difficulty: easy

ingredients

-> Coal distribution: 2/3 below, 1/3 on the lid

- 750g apples
- 100g cranberries
- 5 eggs
- 6 tbsp oatmeal
- 2.5kg potatoes
- 3 tbsp sugar
- 2 onions
- 3 tbsp oil
- salt and pepper

preparation

1.) Preheat the Dutch Oven. Wash and quarter the apples and remove the core. Then cut into narrow strips. Put in the Dutch. Add sugar and 5 tbsp water. Close the lid and bring to the boil. Then stir in the cranberries. Then remove from the coals so that the apple pieces do not disintegrate.

2.) Thoroughly clean the potatoes, then grate them finely with a grater and then squeeze them out on a kitchen towel. Then place in a bowl and add the eggs and mix together. Season to taste with salt.

3.) Peel the onions and rub them with the potato mixture. Taste everything well. Now use the lid of the Dutch oven for frying. To do this, simply add the oil and add the dough you have just made in portions and gradually fry the buffers until golden yellow on both sides. As soon as they are ready, drain them on a kitchen towel and then enjoy with the apple compote.

Crumble with blueberries

KH 47g | EW 5g | F 8g

═══════════════════════════

Preparation time: 20 min + 35 min baking time
Servings: 4
Difficulty: easy

ingredients

-> Coal distribution: 1/3 underneath, 2/3 on the lid

- 500g blueberries / mixed berries
- 100g oatmeal
- 6 tbsp almond flour
- 4 tbsp maple syrup
- 2 tbsp coconut oil
- 1 teaspoon vanilla powder
- 1 tbsp cinnamon
- some salt

preparation

1.) Wash the berries thoroughly under warm water. Do not use hot water or the berries will get mushy. Depending on which berries you prefer, this variety can be selected. After washing, mix with the vanilla powder and 1 tbsp maple syrup.

2.) In a bowl, mix the oat flakes with the almond flour, coconut oil and 1 tbsp maple syrup, so that crumble is formed. Season to taste with salt and cinnamon.

3.) Place the prepared berry mixture in the Dutch Oven on a baking paper and top with the crumble. Close the lid and bake for about 35 minutes until the crumbles take on a brownish color .

KH 40g | EW 16g | F 43g

===

Preparation time: 30 min + 15 min baking time
Servings: 8
Difficulty: easy

ingredients

-> Coal distribution: 1/3 underneath, 2/3 on the lid

- 500g flour
- 300ml warm water
- 40g fresh yeast
- 3 tbsp olive oil
- 2 teaspoons of salt
- 1 teaspoon of sugar
- 2 cups of crème fraîche
- 1 cup of quark
- 250g diced bacon
- 3 onions

preparation

1.) Peel the onions and cut into rings. Then mix the onion rings with the diced bacon and set aside.

2.) Mix the lukewarm water with the yeast and sugar in a bowl, so that a thin dough is formed. Add the flour, olive oil and salt, mix everything thoroughly. If the dough does not come off the edge of the bowl afterwards, simply add a little lukewarm water.

3.) Shape the dough into a ball and let it rise in a warm place until the dough has roughly doubled. Depending on the size of the Dutch oven, roll out the dough whole or in portions. Then dust with plenty of flour and make the topping.

4.) Mix the quark with the crème fraîche in a bowl and season with salt and pepper. Spread both over the dough and pour the onions and pieces of bacon over it. Bake on baking paper over high heat for a few minutes until the dough is crispy.

KH 92g | EW 17g | F 17g

Preparation time: 15 min + 60 min baking time
Servings: 10
Difficulty: easy

ingredients

-> Coal distribution: 1/3 underneath, 2/3 on the lid

- 330g whole wheat flour
- 200g almonds (peeled)
- 200g dried dates
- 200g dried figs
- 200g dried apricots
- 200g dried cranberries
- 150g dried pears
- 7 eggs
- 5 tbsp honey
- 2 teaspoons of gingerbread spice
- 2 teaspoons of cinnamon
- 1 packet of baking powder
- some salt

preparation

1.) Heat the lid of the Dutch Oven and roast the almonds in it. Remove from lid after roasting and transfer to a larger bowl. Chop all the dried fruits and add them to the bowl. The almonds can also be chopped smaller.

2.) Put the eggs in a bowl and beat them with the honey until frothy. Then add the flour, baking powder, gingerbread spice and cinnamon. Mix everything into a smooth dough. Now mix in the nut-fruit mixture you just made.

3.) Line the Dutch Oven with baking paper and preheat. As soon as the Dutch Oven is hot, add the batter. Close the lid and bake for 60 minutes. After about 40 minutes, check whether the bread isn't ready before the set time.

KH 32g | EW 24g | F 29g

Preparation time: 30 min
Servings: 4
Difficulty: easy

ingredients

-> Coal distribution: all briquettes below
- 500ml milk
- 6 eggs
- 1 cup of cream
- some sugar
- some flour

preparation

1.) Put the milk in a bowl and mix with the cream. Separate the eggs and add the yolks to the cream mixture. Beat the egg white with a little sugar until stiff and then add to the mixture. Then add flour until a thick dough is formed.

2.) Use the lid of the Dutch oven and melt some butter in it. Then use a ladle to bake waffles in portions. Then if necessary drain on a kitchen towel and garnish as desired.

KH 50g | EW 7g | F 1g

Preparation time: 135 min + 45 min baking time
Servings: 8
Difficulty: easy

ingredients

-> Coal distribution: 1/3 underneath, 2/3 on the lid

- 435g wheat flour
- 325ml water
- 160g sweet potatoes
- 60g rye flour
- 25g whole wheat flour
- 14g salt
- 1g of fresh yeast

preparation

1.) Peel the sweet potatoes and then grate them finely with a grater. Put aside. Put the flours through a sieve in another bowl. Add the yeast and sweet potatoes and then season with salt. Mix everything together and add the water piece by piece until a smooth dough is formed.

2.) Then take the dough out of the bowl and shape it into a loaf of bread. Cover and let rise in the bowl in a warm place. The dough needs to be stretched at regular intervals. After your dough has risen enough, cut into the top.

3.) Line the Dutch Oven with baking paper and add the loaf of bread. Close the lid and bake for 45 minutes. After 30 minutes, remove the lid to give it a brownish color.

KH 21g | EW 11g | F 24g

===

Preparation time: 20 min + 30 min baking time
Servings: 8
Difficulty: easy

ingredients

-> Coal distribution: 1/3 underneath, 2/3 on the lid

- 225g wheat flour
- 100ml olive oil
- 100ml white wine
- 100g cream cheese
- 100g cooked ham
- 20 pitted green olives
- 20 pitted black olives
- 4 eggs
- 1 tsp baking powder
- some salt

preparation

1.) Mix the flour, the olive oil, the white wine, the eggs and the baking powder in a bowl. Season with a little salt and then mix into a smooth dough.

2.) Cut the ham into small pieces and add to the dough together with the cream cheese. Drain the olives and cut in half. Then put it under the dough.

3.) Shape the finished dough into a loaf of bread and then bake with the lid closed for about 30 minutes until the bread turns brown.

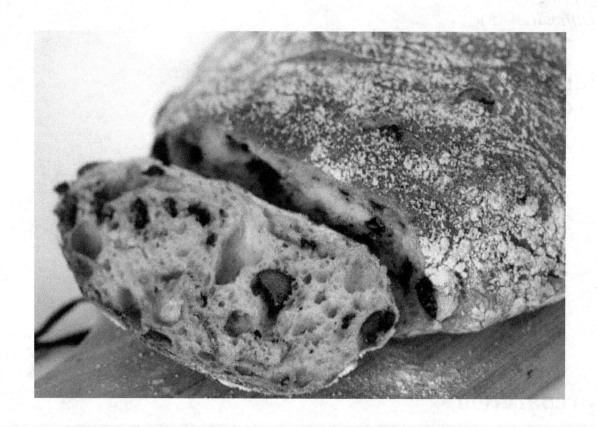

KH 67g | EW 11g | F 13g

===

Preparation time: 90 min + 40 min baking time
Servings: 10
Difficulty: easy

ingredients

-> Coal distribution: 1/3 underneath, 2/3 on the lid
- 750g flour
- 300ml warm milk
- 120g sugar
- 100g butter
- 3 eggs
- 2 tablespoons of cream
- 1 cube of yeast
- some salt

preparation

1.) Heat the milk in a saucepan or the Dutch Oven and then melt the butter in it. As soon as the butter is dissolved, add the yeast and dissolve it too. In another bowl mix the flour, sugar and salt and then stir in the yeast mixture.

2.) Separate the eggs and add everything except 1 egg yolk to the dough. Knead so that a smooth dough is formed for 10 minutes. Cover the bowl and let rise in a warm place for about 1 hour.

3.) Then divide into 8 equal parts and form strands from them and braid the dough into an even braid. Cover again and let rise for 30 minutes. Mix the leftover egg yolk with the cream and use it to generously coat the plait. Then place in the Dutch oven lined with baking paper and bake for 40 minutes.

KH 5g | EW 11g | F 8g

Preparation time: 40 min
Servings: 4
Difficulty: easy

ingredients

-> Coal distribution: all briquettes below

- 250g mushrooms
- 100g onions
- 6 tbsp milk
- 4 eggs
- 2 tbsp parsley
- 2 tbsp olive oil
- salt and pepper

preparation

1.) Peel the onions and then finely chop them. Wash the parsley thoroughly and also chop it into small pieces. Wash the mushrooms and cut into thin slices.

2.) Put the oil in the Dutch Oven and fry the onions until translucent. Add the mushrooms and fry until they have lost a little size. Then season with salt and pepper.

3.) Whisk the eggs with the milk in a bowl and season to taste. Use the lid of the Dutch oven and add oil. Put the egg mixture in the lid and fry until the mixture has thickened and the underside has a brown color. Fill half of the omelette with mushrooms and then fold over. Garnish with the parsley.

KH 69g | EW 12g | F 41g

Preparation time: 30 min + 60 min baking time
Servings: 8
Difficulty: easy

ingredients

-> Coal distribution: 1/3 underneath, 2/3 on the lid

- 750g flour (type 550)
- 450ml of water
- 250g butter
- 100g cream cheese
- 6 tbsp oil
- 1 tbsp honey
- 1 tbsp tomato paste
- 1 cube of yeast
- some salt

preparation

1.) Mix the butter and cream cheese in a bowl. Add the tomato paste and mix everything together thoroughly. Season to taste with the salt.

2.) Now mix the flour with the water in another bowl. Add the oil and add the yeast to the bowl. Mix everything together thoroughly. Season to taste with the honey and salt and knead for 10 minutes.

3.) Roll out the dough and cut into small triangles. Place 3 rectangles on top of each other, each half overlapping, shape into a roll and place in the middle of the Dutch oven lined with baking paper. Drape all other triangles around the middle so that they overlap. Close the lid and bake for about 60 minutes. Check after 45 minutes whether the bread is ready beforehand.

KH 52g | EW 9g | F 5g

Preparation time: 30 min + 60 min baking time
Servings: 8
Difficulty: easy

ingredients

-> Coal distribution: 1/3 underneath, 2/3 on the lid

- 500g spelled flour
- 350ml warm water
- 65g oat flakes (hearty)
- 25g chia seeds
- 2 handfuls of walnut kernels
- 2 tart apples
- 1 tbsp honey
- ½ cube of yeast
- some salt

preparation

1.) Put the warm water in a bowl, add the yeast and dissolve it. Then add the honey to the bowl and let it stand for 10 minutes. In another bowl, mix the flour and oatmeal. Wash the apples thoroughly and then use a grater to grate them finely in the flour. Chop the walnuts and add them.

2.) Add the dissolved yeast mixture to the flour mixture and knead everything together thoroughly. Line the Dutch Oven with parchment paper and pour in the batter. Let it bake for 1 hour, but first check whether the dough is ready earlier. After 15 minutes, make a 2cm cut lengthways. Then finish baking.

Main courses

Rolled roast with mozzarella and mushrooms

KH 35g | EW 101g | F 57g

Preparation time: 40 min + 120 min cooking time
Servings: 6
Difficulty: hard

ingredients

-> Coal distribution: ½ below, ½ on the lid

- 2kg shoulder of a pig
- 200g breadcrumbs
- 250g mushrooms
- 250g mozzarella
- 500ml beef broth
- 500ml vegetable stock
- 250ml dark beer
- 200g crème fraîche
- 2 bundles of soup greens
- salt and pepper
- Spices at will

preparation

1) Cut the pork shoulder into a roulade or have it cut. Mix the breadcrumbs with the spices, distribute thoroughly on the roulade. Leave some space on the outer sides. Cut the mozzarella into slices, wash the mushrooms thoroughly and quarter them. Pour the mixture over the roll roast and tie the whole thing into a roast with butcher's twine.

2) Put a dash of oil in the Dutch Oven. Wash the soup greens thoroughly, cut them into small pieces and then add to the oil. Sear the roll roast and then set it aside. Add the broth, beer and some seasoning to the soup greens, bring everything to the boil and then stir in the crème fraîche.

3) Finally, put the roast back in, close the lid and let the mixture rest for 2 hours. If necessary, add a little broth from time to time. If after 2 hours the sauce is still too thin, thicken it with a sauce thickener. Then puree everything and, if necessary, season again.

Chili con carne

KH 29g | EW 75g | F 50g

===

Preparation time: 40 min +180 min cooking time
Servings: 10
Difficulty: medium

ingredients
-> Coal distribution: 2/3 below, 1/3 on the lid
- 500g bacon
- 3kg beef shanks
- 6 cans of kidney beans
- 2 cans of corn
- 2 cans of pureed tomatoes
- 5 large onions
- 2 cloves of garlic
- 2 tbsp ground coffee
- paprika powder
- Salt and pepper, possibly other spices

preparation

1.) First wash the leg slices and dab them with a paper towel. Then put some olive oil in the Dutch Oven and fry the beef shank slices in it. Divide the bacon 1 or 2 times as desired and also place in the Dutch Oven.

2.) Peel the onion and garlic and cut into small cubes. Add both to the meat and season everything thoroughly. After a few minutes, add the tomatoes and the coffee so that the meat does not burn.

3.) Let the whole simmer for about 3 hours until the meat falls off the bone and the pulp is cooked out. Then drain the beans and corn. Add both to the meat and stir thoroughly. Season again if necessary.

4.) Now put some briquettes on the lid so that toasted aromas develop. The chilli is ready after about 2-3 hours. Now only the bone has to be removed.

KH 6g | EW 50g | F 53g

==

Preparation time: 40 min
Servings: 4
Difficulty: medium

ingredients
-> Coal distribution: 1/3 under the pot, 2/3 on the lid
- 150g walnuts
- 900g wild salmon
- 1 bunch of parsley
- 3 tbsp breadcrumbs
- 3 tbsp parmesan (grated)
- 100g butter
- 1 lemon
- salt and pepper

preparation

1.) Wash the lemon thoroughly under hot water until the smell comes out. Then wash the wild salmon as well and pat dry with a kitchen towel. Season to taste with the lemon juice and add salt and pepper.

2.) Wash the parsley thoroughly and chop it together with the walnuts. Then knead with the breadcrumbs, parmesan and butter in a bowl and season to taste.

3.) Lightly oil the Dutch Oven and then add the wild salmon. Spread the mixture generously on the salmon and press down a little.

4.) Finally just put the lid on and let the salmon cook in peace until the salmon is juicy with a nutty crust.

KH 56g | EW 20g | F 43g

===

Preparation time: 60 min
Servings: 4
Difficulty: easy

ingredients

-> Coal distribution: 1/3 underneath, 2/3 on the lid
- 1 loaf of brown bread
- 100g Emmentaler
- 100g bacon
- 1 clove of garlic
- 5 tbsp olive oil
- ½ bunch of parsley
- ½ bunch of chives

preparation

1.) First peel the garlic and then finely chop it. Wash the chives and parsley thoroughly and also chop them into small pieces. Mix all ingredients with the oil.

2.) Take the brown bread and cut into a diamond shape down to the bottom. First put a slice of the Emmentaler in the slit that has been created. Now brush the bread generously with the oil mixture. Cut the bacon into small cubes and pour over the coated bread.

3.) Put the garnished bread in the preheated Dutch Oven and let it bake for 35 minutes.

4.) Then take it out, let it cool down briefly and don't allow too much time to pass before consumption so that the cheese is still melted.

Vegetable quiche

KH 35g | EW 23g | F 36g

Preparation time: 70 min + 45 min cooking time
Servings: 6
Difficulty: medium

ingredients
-> Coal distribution: 1/3 underneath, 2/3 on the lid

- 6 eggs
- 250g flour
- 1 cauliflower
- 350g carrots
- 100g butter
- 2 onions
- 1 bell pepper
- 200ml vegetable stock
- 200g peas
- 1 tbsp olive oil
- 150g grated Gouda cheese
- 100g whipped cream
- salt and pepper

preparation

1.) Mix the flour, 1 egg, 1 teaspoon salt, butter and 4 teaspoons of water. Wrap in foil and put in the fridge for 30 minutes. Remove and wash the cauliflower florets. Peel the onions, wash the peppers, cut both into small cubes. Put some olive oil in the Dutch Oven and sauté the onions and florets in it.

2.) Boil the mixture with the broth and simmer for 10 minutes. Peel the carrots and cut them into small cubes. Place in the Dutch oven with the peas and bell pepper. As soon as the carrots are firm to the bite, set the vegetables aside.

3.) Brush the Dutch Oven with oil, roll out the dough and use a fork to perforate the base. Put the vegetable filling on top and sprinkle with cheese. Mix together 5 eggs, cream and spices in a bowl and pour over. Pour cheese over it again, close the lid and bake for 45 minutes.

KH 57g | EW 29g | F 21g

Preparation time: 30 min + 35 min cooking time
Servings: 8
Difficulty: medium

ingredients

-> Coal distribution: 1/3 underneath, 2/3 on the lid

- 1 pack of lasagne sheets
- 2 packs of spinach leaves (frozen)
- 2 packs of creamed spinach (frozen)
- 800ml milk
- 4 packages of cream cheese
- 2 cloves of garlic
- 1 package of grated cheese of your choice
- salt and pepper

preparation

1.) First put the milk in the Dutch Oven and heat it up. Then add the cream cheese and let it dissolve.

2.) Let the spinach thaw, wash and dry. Then add to the milk mass and simmer. Taste everything.

3.) Peel the garlic and dice it, also add to the mixture. If necessary, you can leave this out. After a few minutes of simmering, transfer the mixture to another container.

4.) Place the first layer of lasagne sheets in the empty Dutch Oven and distribute them evenly. Then pour the mixture and repeat this process until the mixture is completely used up and the last layer consists of the mixture.

5.) Now spread the cheese generously over the last layer and then bake in the Dutch oven for 35 minutes. Important: because of the spinach, only serve the lasagna cold the next day.

Pumpkin curry

KH 46g | EW 13g | F 1g

═══════════════════════════════

Preparation time: 20 min + 35 min cooking time
Servings: 3
Difficulty: easy

ingredients
-> Coal distribution: all briquettes below
- 1 Hokkaido pumpkin
- 1 piece of ginger as you like
- 100g red lentils
- 2 hands full of cranberries
- 1 clove of garlic
- 1 onion
- 500ml vegetable stock
- 2 teaspoons of curry spice
- 1 tbsp tomato paste
- 2 tbsp oil
- salt and pepper

preparation

1.) Remove the flesh of the pumpkin from the pumpkin so that the bowl can be used as a bowl for serving. Cut the removed meat into cubes.

2.) Peel and chop the onions, garlic and ginger. Then sweat the cubes in the through oven with a little oil. Add the tomato paste and mix everything thoroughly. After everything has got a good color, deglaze with the vegetable stock.

3.) Round off with the lentils, cranberries and curry powder and simmer for 10 minutes. Finally, add the pumpkin so that it doesn't get too soft. Then simmer for another 15 minutes. As soon as the curry is ready, serve in the hollowed out pumpkin.

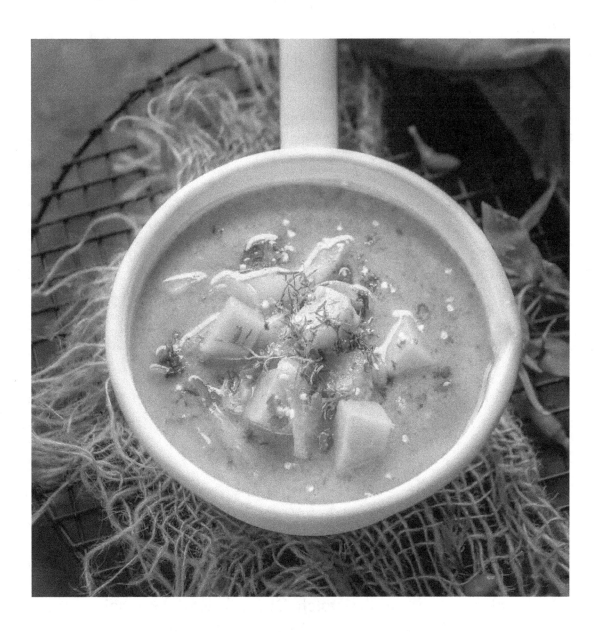

KH 53g | EW 32g | F 3g

===============

Preparation time: 20 min + 90 min cooking time
Servings: 3
Difficulty: easy

ingredients

-> Coal distribution: all briquettes on the lid

- 2 large squids
- 5 large potatoes
- 5 tomatoes
- 1 onion
- 1 clove of garlic
- Mediterranean herbs

preparation

1.) Thoroughly clean the potatoes and then peel them. Then cut into even columns. In the Dutch Oven, lightly fry the potato wedges with a little oil and season a little.

2.) Wash the tomatoes thoroughly, remove the stalk and dice them. Peel and finely chop the onion and garlic. Add to the potato wedges in the Dutch Oven and simmer.

3.) Put the squids with the arms upwards in the pot and then place the lid on the Dutch Oven. Season the whole thing with the Mediterranean herbs. Now let the mixture simmer for about 90 minutes.

KH 14g | EW 62g | F 33g

Preparation time: 30 min + 160 min cooking time
Servings: 8
Difficulty: medium

ingredients

-> Coal distribution: 1/3 underneath, 2/3 on the lid

- 2kg ribs
- ribs spice
- 600ml orange juice
- 4 tbsp Worcester sauce
- 2 tbsp balsamic vinegar
- 2 tbsp soy sauce
- 2 teaspoons of ginger
- 2 tbsp garlic
- 5 tbsp brown sugar
- 5 tbsp honey
- 1 tsp chilli (chopped)
- 3 teaspoons of cinnamon

preparation

1.) Rub the ribs with the rib spice the day before and leave to rest in the refrigerator overnight.

2.) The next day, melt the butter in the Dutch Oven and spread the ribs on the bottom. Mix the orange juice, Worcester sauce, balsamic vinegar, soy sauce, brown sugar, honey, cinnamon and chilli together. Peel and chop ginger and garlic. Spread all the ingredients over the ribs.

3.) After an hour, turn the ribs so that all ribs are well marinated. Skim off most of the sauce after 2 hours. Place a stainless steel container in the Dutch Oven, place a grid on it and distribute the ribs on it.

4.) Double the briquettes. Let the sauce thicken and glaze the ribs with it. Then bake for 35 minutes.

KH 12g | EW 11g | F 22g

====================

Preparation time: 30 min + 20 min cooking time
Servings: 6
Difficulty: easy

ingredients

-> Coal distribution: ½ underneath, ½ on the lid

- 200g bacon
- 250g white beans
- 250g red beans
- 200g tomatoes
- 2 onions
- 2 cloves of garlic
- 2 tbsp tomato paste
- 1 tbsp honey
- 80ml beef broth
- 2 tbsp olive oil
- salt and pepper

preparation

1.) Pour the two beans through a sieve and allow them to drain. Then rinse with cold water. Peel the onions and garlic and chop both into small pieces. Cut the bacon into small cubes.

2.) Wash the tomatoes thoroughly and remove the stalk. Then roll the dice. Preheat the Dutch oven and add a little olive oil. Fry the bacon, garlic and onions in the oil.

3.) Then mix in the beans, tomato paste and honey and season thoroughly with salt and pepper. Finally, mix the tomatoes with the other ingredients and add the beef broth.

4.) Close the lid and bring the bean pot to a boil. If necessary, taste again after 10 minutes and mix well.

KH 51g | EW 35g | F 33g

═══════════════════════════

Preparation time: 20 min + 25 baking time
Servings: 4
Difficulty: easy

ingredients

-> Coal distribution: all briquettes below
- 1 finished pizza dough
- 1 pack of herbal cream cheese
- 5 fresh tomatoes
- 2 packs of mozzarella
- fresh basil
- 1 packet of grated pizza cheese
- salt and pepper

preparation

1.) The lid of the Dutch oven is used for this recipe. Grease the lid and cover with flour. Roll out the dough evenly on the floured lid and brush with the cream cheese.

2.) Wash the tomatoes thoroughly, remove the stalk and cut into even slices. Drain the mozzarella and cut into thin slices. Spread the tomatoes, mozzarella and basil on the pizza. Season the topping and cover completely with the pizza cheese.

3.) Spread the briquettes and let the pizza bake for 25 minutes. Of course, the pizza can be topped with any ingredients as you like.

KH 22g | EW 47g | F 69g

Preparation time: 30 min + 180 min cooking time
Servings: 12
Difficulty: easy

ingredients

-> Coal distribution: 1/3 underneath, 2/3 on the lid
- 3kg pork neck
- 400g bacon
- 250g BBQ rub
- 500ml BBQ sauce
- 4 large vegetable onions
- 2 large peppers

preparation

1.) Cut the neck of the pork into 1cm thick slices the day before and remove the bone if necessary. Then smear the slices generously with the rub and then put them in the fridge overnight, wrapping them well.

2.) The next day, peel the onion, core the peppers and remove the stalk. Cut both into thin slices.

3.) Line the bottom of the Dutch oven with the bacon. Then add a layer of meat to the bacon layer and then put another layer of the onions and peppers. Repeat this layering process until all the ingredients have been used. Cover the whole thing with BBQ sauce and finish with a checkerboard pattern made of bacon. Put the lid on the pot and let the layered meat cook for 3 hours.

KH 9g | EW 31g | F 12g

═══════════════════════════════════════

Preparation time: 30 min + 90 min cooking time
Servings: 6
Difficulty: easy

ingredients

-> Coal distribution: 1/2 below, 1/2 on the lid

- 900g roast beef
- 5 onions
- 2 cloves of garlic
- 1 bottle of red wine
- 2 bay leaves
- 2 tbsp olive oil
- 1/2 teaspoon cinnamon
- 1/2 teaspoon cloves (ground)
- 1 teaspoon of caraway seeds
- 3 tbsp tomato paste
- salt and pepper

preparation

1.) First peel the onions and the garlic cloves and chop them into small pieces. Then add a little oil to the preheated Dutch oven and let it simmer.

2.) Dice the meat as well, proceeding a little coarser or finer depending on your preference, then add to the onions and garlic in the Dutch oven. As soon as the meat has turned brown on all sides, season with the cinnamon, cloves and caraway seeds.

3.) Stir in the tomato paste and season with salt and pepper. Finally, pour in the red wine and add the bay leaves. Always be careful that nothing burns on the floor. As soon as all the ingredients are in the Dutch Oven, close the lid and let simmer for about 90 minutes.

KH 21g | EW 24g | F 22g

========

Preparation time: 30 min + 120 min cooking time
Servings: 8
Difficulty: medium

ingredients

-> Coal distribution: 1/2 below, 1/2 on the lid

- 1kg of beef
- 400g onions
- 1 pineapple
- 2 tbsp vegetable oil
- 2 tbsp clarified butter
- 1 chili
- Curry powder of your choice
- salt and pepper

preparation

1.) Take the meat and dice it into bite-sized pieces. As soon as all the meat has been diced, drizzle with the vegetable oil and season with the curry powder, salt and pepper as desired.

2.) Peel the onions thoroughly and then dice them into small pieces. Remove the peel from the pineapple, remove the stalk and cut the pulp into small cubes. Wash the chilli thoroughly and remove the seeds if necessary. Then also divide into small pieces.

3.) Put the clarified butter in the Dutch Oven and heat it up. Add the pieces of meat and fry them. Then add the onions and the chilli pieces. As soon as the onions are translucent, add the pineapple cubes and some water to the Dutch oven and simmer for about 2 hours with the lid closed. To prevent the curry from burning, it is best to stir constantly and, if necessary, add new water.

Potatoes with meat in the pot

KH 42g | EW 20g | F 15g

===

Preparation time: 30 min + 180 min cooking time
Servings: 10
Difficulty: easy

ingredients
-> Coal distribution: 1/2 below, 1/2 on the lid
- 600g smoked pork
- 1.5kg potatoes
- 600g onions
- 200g Mettenden
- 1kg of carrots
- 300ml white wine
- 200g crème fraîche
- 5 tablespoons of broth (granular)
- 4 tablespoons rapeseed oil
- 6 sprigs of thyme
- salt and pepper

preparation

1.) Remove the skin from the onions and then dice them into small pieces. Wash, peel and cut the carrots. Clean the potatoes and cut into cubes. Put all ingredients aside for now.

2.) Cut the meatloaf and cut the smoked pork into cubes. Wash the thyme and separate the leaves from the branches.

3.) Put a little oil in the Dutch Oven and fry the meatloaf and the smoked pork with the thyme. After searing, layer the previously cut ingredients on the smoked pork and finish with a layer of potatoes. Season everything thoroughly with salt and pepper.

4.) Thoroughly mix the white wine with 750ml water and the broth in a bowl. Pour the mixture over the layers and then simmer for 3 hours. The crème fraîche can be used for serving.

KH 17g | EW 30g | F 18g

Preparation time: 30 min + 30 min cooking time
Servings: 6
Difficulty: easy

ingredients

-> Coal distribution: 2/3 below, 1/3 on the lid

- 250g smoked sausage of your choice
- 200g ready-to-eat crabs
- 250g ham (lean)
- 1 1/2 cups of rice
- 3 tomatoes
- 3 onions
- 1 bell pepper
- 2 cloves of garlic
- 2 bay leaves
- 1 pepper
- olive oil

preparation

1.) Peel the onions and garlic cloves and then dice them into small pieces. Also cut the lean ham and smoked sausage into small pieces.

2.) Put a little oil in the Dutch Oven and fry the onion and garlic cubes in it. As soon as the onions are translucent, add the sausage and ham and fry them.

3.) Wash the tomatoes thoroughly, peel, remove the stalk and dice. Then also put in the Dutch Oven. Wash the peppers, remove the seeds and the stalk and cut into small pieces. Then also add to the pot.

4.) Wash the rice thoroughly in a sieve until the water is clear and then add 3 cups of water to the mixture. Round off the whole thing with the pepper and bay leaves and simmer for about 15 minutes. Finally, after 15 minutes, add the crabs to the jambalaya and simmer for another 15 minutes.

Cauliflower risotto with minced meat

KH 29g | EW 28g | F 25g

Preparation time: 40 min + 30 min cooking time
Servings: 8
Difficulty: medium

ingredients

-> Coal distribution: 2/3 below, 1/3 on the lid
- 600g ground beef
- 200g risotto rice
- 150g parmesan cheese
- 7 tomatoes
- 3 onions
- 2 cauliflowers
- 2 cloves of garlic
- olive oil
- beef broth

preparation

1.) Peel and dice the onions. Remove the cauliflower florets from the stalk and wash thoroughly. Put a little oil in the Dutch Oven and fry the minced meat in it.

2.) Peel the garlic and place in the Dutch Oven together with the diced onions and sauté. Taste everything well. Wash the tomatoes thoroughly, remove the stalk and dice. Add the tomatoes with the risotto rice and the cauliflower to the minced meat.

3.) Now fill the Dutch Oven with enough broth. Close the lid and let it cook until the cauliflower is firm to the bite. Just before the end, add the parmesan.

Cheese noodles

KH 45g | EW 17g | F 26g

═══════════════════════════

Preparation time: 30 min + 20 min cooking time
Servings: 4
Difficulty: easy

ingredients

-> Coal distribution: 1/3 underneath, 2/3 on the lid

- 600g spaetzle
- 150g Gouda (grated)
- 3 onions
- 3 tbsp oil
- 3 tbsp flour
- salt and pepper

preparation

1.) Put water in the Dutch Oven and season with salt. Add the spaetzle and cook for about 12 minutes. Peel the onions and divide them into individual rings. Then turn them in flour.

2.) After the spaetzle have finished cooking, drain them through a sieve. Pour the oil into the empty Dutch Oven and sauté the onion rings until they turn golden brown.

3.) Then add the spaetzle and add the cheese to everything. Mix well and bake for about 15 minutes.

KH 29g | EW 6g | F 11g

======================================

Preparation time: 70 min + 10 min cooking time
Servings: 8
Difficulty: easy

ingredients

-> Coal distribution: 2/3 below, 1/3 on the lid

- 1.2 liters of vegetable stock
- 400g mushrooms
- 400g carrots
- 300g rice
- 6 tbsp olive oil
- 3 tbsp soy sauce
- 3 bananas
- 1 Chinese cabbage
- 1 bunch of spring onions
- 1 lemon

preparation

1.) Put the vegetable stock in the Dutch Oven and bring to the boil. Add the rice and let it soak for about 40 minutes on a not so high heat.

2.) Thoroughly clean the spring onions, carrots and mushrooms and then cut everything into thin slices. Immediately drizzle the mushrooms with the lemon juice from half a lemon.

3.) Peel the bananas and cut them into slices. Heat 3 tablespoons of oil in the lid of the Dutch Oven and sauté all previously cut ingredients. Stir continuously for 10 minutes so that nothing burns.

4.) Remove some leaves from the Chinese cabbage and wash them thoroughly and then cut them into strips. Now add the leaves and the contents of the lid to the rice in the Dutch Oven, mix everything thoroughly and season if necessary. Let everything cook together for 10 minutes with the lid closed.

KH 26g | EW 46g | F 34g

===

Preparation time: 40 min + 75 min cooking time
Servings: 10
Difficulty: easy

ingredients

-> Coal distribution: 1/3 underneath, 2/3 on the lid

- 1.6kg of chicken
- 250g flour
- 250ml brandy
- 250g clarified butter
- 250g mushrooms
- 100g rib bacon
- 5 carrots
- 5 onions
- 1 bottle of Beaujolais
- salt and pepper

preparation

1.) Divide the chicken into individual portions. Remove the skin completely. Wash and pat the meat. Preheat the Dutch Oven, then add the wine and bring to the boil until it has reduced by half.

2.) Season the meat and roll it in a bowl with flour. Now use the lid of the Dutch oven and dissolve butter in it. Sear the meat that was previously turned in flour.

3.) Peel the carrots and onions and dice them. Dice the bacon. Fry everything in the lid and then place in the Dutch Oven. Season everything to taste and top up with the brandy. Close the lid and let cook for 1 hour.

4.) At the end of the cooking time, remove the lid, season again if necessary and then melt clarified butter in the lid and fry the previously washed and cut mushrooms. Then add to the Dutch oven for a few minutes and serve.

KH 43g | EW 34g | F 33g

Preparation time: 30 min + 45 min cooking time
Servings: 10
Difficulty: medium

ingredients

-> Coal distribution: ½ underneath, ½ on the lid

- 1.5kg ground beef
- 1.5kg potatoes (waxy)
- 4 onions
- 1 head of white cabbage
- 200ml cream
- 1 bunch of soup vegetables
- 3 eggs
- 3 tbsp mustard
- cornstarch
- lard
- bread flour
- salt and pepper

preparation

1.) Bring the water to the boil in the Dutch Oven. Salt and cook the cabbage in it. Peel the onions, wash the parsley, chop both into small pieces. Knead the eggs, mustard, parsley and minced meat together. Add the breadcrumbs.

2.) Take the cabbage head out of the Dutch Oven, loosen the leaves and remove the stem. Spread the minced meat mixture on top and form into packages. Fix the packages with a piece of kitchen twine.

3.) Wash the soup vegetables and cut them into small pieces. Brush the Dutch oven with the lard and dissolve in it. Fry the cabbage mince packets on all sides in the dissolved lard.

4.) Put the soup greens and the onions in the Dutch Oven and sauté. After 7 minutes, deglaze everything with water and simmer for about 45 minutes. Wash and chop the potatoes. 25 minutes before the end of the cooking time, add the potatoes to the saucepan and bring to the boil with the cream.

KH 29g | EW 7g | F 3g

===

Preparation time: 30 min + 30 min cooking time
Servings: 8
Difficulty: easy

ingredients

-> Coal distribution: 1/3 underneath, 2/3 on the lid

- 600g potatoes
- 500ml vegetable stock
- 400g tofu
- 300g corn
- 25g ginger
- 4 cloves of garlic
- 3 zucchinis
- 2 onions
- 2 tbsp coconut oil
- 1 green chilli pepper
- 1 can of coconut milk
- Spices at will

preparation

1.) Peel the onions, garlic and ginger and chop everything. Core the chilli pepper and cut into small rings. Clean the potatoes, remove the skin and dice. Drain the tofu and then also cut into cubes.

2.) Preheat the Dutch Oven and fry the onions, garlic, ginger and chilli in it. As soon as the onions are translucent, add the tofu until it has a brownish color. Then add the potato cubes and deglaze with the broth. Then let everything simmer for 15 minutes.

3.) Wash the zucchini, remove the ends and cut into slices. Drain the corn and place in the Dutch Oven with the zucchini strips and coconut milk and simmer for another 15 minutes. Season with spices to taste.

KH 33g | EW 24g | F 17g

================

Preparation time: 30 min + 60 min cooking time
Servings: 4
Difficulty: easy

ingredients

-> Coal distribution: ½ underneath, ½ on the lid

- 500g duck breast
- 2 cloves of garlic
- 1 pineapple
- 1 onion
- 1 can of tomatoes (peeled)
- 1 teaspoon ginger (grated)
- 1 tbsp curry powder
- 1 tbsp sugar
- 1 tbsp vinegar
- 2 tbsp oil
- salt and pepper

preparation

1.) First separate the skin from the duck breast and then cut both into strips. Preheat the Dutch oven and then add the oil. Fry both the duck and the meat in the hot oil.

2.) Remove the peel from the pineapple and remove the stalk. Quarter the pineapple and add to the meat together with the tomatoes. Peel and chop the onions and garlic. Then also add to the Dutch oven.

3.) Now season everything with the vinegar, the sugar, the curry powder and the ginger. Mix everything together thoroughly and add salt and pepper. Now close the lid and let it cook for about 1 hour.

KH 41g | EW 15g | F 12g

========

Preparation time: 25 min + 60 min cooking time
Servings: 8
Difficulty: easy

ingredients

-> Coal distribution: ½ underneath, ½ on the lid

- 400g whole wheat pasta
- 300g ground beef
- 800ml canned tomatoes
- 2 onions
- 2 carrots
- 2 celery
- 2 tbsp olive oil
- 2 teaspoons of dried oregano
- 1 clove of garlic
- 1 chilli pepper
- salt and pepper

preparation

1.) Preheat the Dutch Oven. Peel and chop the onions and garlic. As soon as the Dutch Oven is preheated add the olive oil. Add the onions and garlic to the oil and sauté in it until translucent. Peel the carrots and clean the celery. Cut both into small pieces.

2.) Add the minced meat to the onions and cut into small pieces. After about 5 minutes add the carrots and celery to the minced meat. Add the oregano to everything. After another 5 minutes, pour the canned tomatoes on top. Close the lid and let everything cook. Stir every 15 minutes. If there is not enough water, add a little water. The Bolognese is ready as soon as the mince is no longer pink and the vegetables have a firm consistency.

3.) Cook the pasta in lightly salted water in advance until the pasta is firm to the bite. Either use the Dutch Oven or another pot if necessary.

KH 70g | EW 34g | F 55g

=======

Preparation time: 60 min + 35 min cooking time
Servings: 6
Difficulty: easy

ingredients

-> Coal distribution: 1/3 underneath, 2/3 on the lid

- 500g macaroni
- 200g cheddar
- 200g Emmentaler
- 100g parmesan cheese
- 400ml milk
- 200ml cream
- 90g butter
- 50g breadcrumbs
- 40g flour
- 1 clove of garlic
- salt and pepper

preparation

1.) Heat the Dutch Oven. Heat 60g butter in it and clarify, then remove the Dutch Oven from the coals and use a whisk to stir the flour into the butter until it becomes smooth.

2.) Then slowly add the milk and cream and bring to the boil, stirring constantly. Season to taste and simmer over low heat for 10 minutes.

3.) Cook the macaroni in a little salted water until they are firm to the bite. Then add the cheeses to the saucepan. Mix everything thoroughly until you get a tough mixture. If necessary, season again.

4.) Peel the garlic and put it through a garlic press. Now heat the lid of the Dutch oven and melt 30g butter in it. Toast the breadcrumbs with the garlic until the breadcrumbs are lightly browned. Then spread the macaroni on the cheese and bake with the lid closed in the Dutch oven for about 35 minutes until the surface is golden brown.

KH 38g | EW 23g | F 9g

═══════════════════════════════════

Preparation time: 40 min + 30 min cooking time
Servings: 8
Difficulty: easy

ingredients

-> Coal distribution: 1/3 underneath, 2/3 on the lid

- 500g potatoes
- 500g redfish fillet
- 500g tomatoes cut into pieces
- 1 pack of frozen spinach
- 1 lemon
- 150g Emmentaler (grated)
- 250g breadcrumbs
- some butter
- salt and pepper

preparation

1.) Preheat the Dutch Oven and then add the butter. Peel the potatoes and then cut them into slices and line the base of the Dutch oven with them. Add a little water and let it soften. Then spread the spinach over it and season everything well.

2.) Wash the lemon under hot water and then drizzle the lemon juice over the fish. Place on top of the spinach and then the tomato pieces over the fish. Mix the grated cheese with the breadcrumbs in a bowl and cover the fish with them.

3.) Now spread a few more flakes of butter over it and then bake for about 30 minutes. Test beforehand whether the fish is not ready. Then season again to taste.

KH 11g | EW 83g | F 43g

Preparation time: 30 min + 180 min cooking time
Servings: 6
Difficulty: easy

ingredients

-> Coal distribution: ½ underneath, ½ on the lid

- 2kg ribs
- 5 stalks of celery
- 3 medium hot chillies
- 3 carrots
- 5 shallots
- 3 cloves of garlic
- 4 teaspoons sweet chili sauce
- mustard
- 1 bottle of ginger ale
- 1 small ginger bulb
- 500ml vegetable stock
- salt and pepper

preparation

1.) Rub the ribs thoroughly with the selected mustard one day before preparation, season to taste and then leave to steep overnight.

2.) Preheat the Dutch Oven the following day. Wash and dice the shallots. Now place the ribs in the Dutch Oven and fry them briefly. Then remove and fry the shallots in the fat of the ribs. Peel the garlic and ginger, wash the chillies. Chop everything into small pieces, add to the saucepan and stir well.

3.) Then deglaze with the ginger ale and let it boil down. Then pour in half of the vegetable stock and put the ribs back into the pot. Cover and cook for 2 hours.

4.) Peel the carrots, wash the celery and cut both into slices. After the 2 hours put in the Dutch Oven and season with the sweet chili sauce. Then cook again for 1 hour.

KH 17g | EW 14g | F 13g

Preparation time: 30 min + 35 min cooking time
Servings: 6
Difficulty: easy

ingredients

-> Coal distribution: 2/3 below, 1/3 on the lid

- 6 peppers (choose color as you like)
- 10 large mushrooms
- 200g mixed minced meat
- 1 large onion
- 2 cloves of garlic
- 5 tbsp oil
- 200g cooked rice
- 250ml tomato sauce
- 100g cheddar (grated)
- salt and pepper

preparation

1.) Preheat the Dutch Oven. Peel the onions and garlic, add a little oil to the Dutch oven and sauté until translucent. Wash the peppers thoroughly. Carefully remove the lid and remove the seeds. Put the hollowed out peppers and the removed lids aside.

2.) Now add the minced meat to the garlic and onions in the Dutch Oven. Wash and dice the mushrooms. Also add. Now put the rice in the pot, fry everything well and mix.

3.) Stir in half of the tomato sauce, season everything to taste and remove from the Dutch oven as soon as everything is ready. Now fill the wrapped peppers with the filling you just made and place them well in the Dutch Oven.

4.) Distribute the remaining tomato sauce evenly on the filled peppers, garnish with the cheddar and then put the lid of the peppers on top. Let it cook for 25 minutes with the lid closed.

KH 21g | EW 35g | F 50g

Preparation time: 20 min + 90 min baking time
Servings: 6
Difficulty: easy

ingredients

-> Coal distribution: 1/3 underneath, 2/3 on the lid

- 800g ground beef
- 150g Emmentaler (grated)
- 6 large mushrooms
- 4 large potatoes
- 3 tbsp BBQ rub
- 2 tbsp herbs of Provence
- 1 packet of bacon
- 1 clove of garlic
- 1 bottle of Cremefine
- some oil
- salt and pepper

preparation

1.) Preheat the Dutch Oven and then add the oil. Now line the base with 4 slices of bacon. Season the minced meat well. Wash the mushrooms thoroughly and cut them into slices. Peel and chop the garlic.

2.) Peel the potatoes and cut into slices. Now layer the individual components. Start with the hack and spread the BBQ rub over it. Pour the mushrooms over it and then spread the garlic.

3.) Repeat this layering until the last layer is potatoes. is completed. Season the potato layers thoroughly with salt, pepper and Provence herbs.

4.) Pour the Cremefine over the last layer of potatoes and cover the whole with the Emmentaler. Finally, spread the bacon over it and then bake with the lid closed for about 90 minutes.

KH 27g | EW 35g | F 35g

==

Preparation time: 80 min + 150 min cooking time
Servings: 8
Difficulty easy

ingredients

-> **Coal distribution: 1/3 underneath, 2/3 on the lid**

- 700ml beef broth
- 500g white beans
- 400g canned tomatoes
- 300g bacon in one piece
- 250g tomato ketchup
- 150g onions
- 100g brown sugar
- 100ml orange juice
- 50g sugar
- 6 chicken wings
- 6 chicken legs
- 2 tbsp honey
- 1 tbsp chili powder
- salt and pepper

preparation

1.) Preheat the Dutch Oven. Peel and chop the onions. Put the beans in a colander and wash them off. Cut the bacon into slices and sauté with the onions in the Dutch oven. Add the beans and brown sugar, stir-fry for 3 minutes. Deglaze with the tomatoes,

600ml beef stock and 150ml of the ketchup and simmer for 2 hours.

2.) After 2 hours, remove the lid and let it simmer until the sauce becomes thick. To taste. Mix the orange juice with the chili powder, honey, sugar and ketchup. Rinse and pat the chicken wings and legs, then brush the marinade thoroughly. Let it steep for 60 minutes. Then put some oil in the lid of the Dutch oven and fry the chicken legs in it. As soon as all the legs are ready, add them to the bean mixture.

KH 66g | EW 45g | F 42g

===

Preparation time: 40 min + 45 min baking time
Servings: 6
Difficulty: easy

ingredients

-> Coal distribution: 1/3 underneath, 2/3 on the lid

- 1kg ground beef
- 1kg of potatoes
- 400g canned tomatoes (pieces)
- 3 cloves of garlic
- 3 eggplants
- 90g parmesan
- 40g butter
- 40g flour
- 400ml milk
- 1 large onion
- 1 pinch of cinnamon
- some olive oil
- salt and pepper

preparation

1.) Pre-cook the potatoes. Then peel, cut into even slices and season. Wash the aubergines and slice 2 of them , the third lengthways. Mix a marinade with oil, salt and pepper and pickle the aubergines. In the preheated lid of the pot, fry the aubergines with a little oil. Peel and finely chop the onion and garlic, add to the pan and fry with the mince.

2.) Add the tomatoes, season to taste and simmer until the liquid has evaporated. Grease the Dutch Oven and line the edge with aubergine strips. Now layer the potatoes, aubergines and minced meat. Melt the butter for the sauce. Add the flour, milk and parmesan until you get a smooth sauce. Season to taste and let steep for 10 minutes . Pour over the layers and bake for 45 minutes with the lid closed.

KH 25g | EW 20g | F 7g

===

Preparation time: 30 min + 45 min cooking time
Servings: 4
Difficulty: medium

ingredients
-> Coal distribution: 1/3 underneath, 2/3 on the lid
- 2 legs of lamb
- 400ml lamb stock
- 200ml red wine
- 1kg of chunky tomatoes
- 3 cloves of garlic
- 5 carrots
- 1 leek
- 3 onions
- 2 tbsp herbs of Provence
- some cane sugar
- oil
- salt and pepper

preparation

1.) Make a marinade from the herbs, salt and cane sugar in a bowl and use it to marinate the legs of lamb thoroughly.

2.) Peel and chop the garlic cloves. Peel and chop the onions as well. Put both in the Dutch Oven with a little oil and let fry. Peel the carrots, remove the ends and then cut into thin slices. Wash the leek and cut into small pieces. Put both in the Dutch Oven as soon as the onions are lightly steamed.

3.) Now put the chunky tomatoes in the pot and bed the leg of lamb on the vegetables. Then add the red wine and lamb stock. Close the lid and let everything stew for 45 minutes. After about 30 minutes, check whether the legs of lamb are not ready beforehand.

KH 51g | EW 12g | F 4g

==

Preparation time: 80 min
Servings: 6
Difficulty: easy

ingredients

-> Coal distribution: 1/3 underneath, 2/3 on the lid

- 600g eggplant
- 500g sweet potatoes
- 300ml vegetable stock
- 300g yogurt
- 240g chickpeas
- 60g raisins
- 20g ginger
- 1 clove of garlic
- 1 can of coconut milk
- 1 can of chopped tomatoes
- 2 limes
- salt and pepper

preparation

1.) Preheat the Dutch Oven. Wash the aubergines, dice them, season them well and then let them steep for 30 minutes. Peel and finely chop the garlic, onions and ginger. Sauté the onions, garlic and ginger in a little oil until the onions are translucent. Add the raisins and pour the coconut milk, tomatoes and broth on top. Simmer for 20 minutes.

2.) Meanwhile, peel and dice the sweet potatoes. Puree everything in the pot after the 20 minutes. Now fry the aubergine with a little oil in the lid of the Dutch oven. Wash the chickpeas in a sieve and then dry them off. Then put the sweet potatoes in the Dutch Oven, simmer for 30 minutes and then refine with the juice of a lime.

3.) For the topping, wash the other lime thoroughly and use the grater to rub the peel and mix it with the yogurt. Then add the juice and season to taste.

KH 46g | EW 12g | F 6g

═══════════════════════════════

Preparation time: 70 min
Servings: 4
Difficulty: medium

ingredients

-> Coal distribution: 1/3 underneath, 2/3 on the lid

- 500g asparagus (green)
- 200g risotto rice
- 100ml white wine
- 100g rocket
- 6 tbsp parmesan
- 7 tbsp olive oil
- 4 tbsp pine nuts
- 1 liter of vegetable stock
- 1 onion
- 1 clove of garlic

preparation

1.) Heat salted water in the Dutch Oven. Wash the asparagus, remove the ends and add to the water for 7 minutes. Rinse after cooking and cut into slices.

2.) Peel and chop the onion and garlic. Put 1 tablespoon of olive oil in the Dutch Oven and sauté the onions until translucent. Add the garlic and risotto rice and sauté for 3 minutes. Now pour a ladle of vegetable stock over the rice, close the lid and let it simmer. As soon as the rice has soaked up the liquid, pour another ladle with the vegetable stock over it until the vegetable stock is completely used up. Also add the white wine.

3.) As soon as the rice is ready, remove the lid of the Dutch oven and use it as a pan to roast the pine nuts. Wash the rocket and pat dry. Then chop up. Now mix the pine nuts, the asparagus, the rocket, the remaining olive oil and the parmesan into the rice and mix everything together.

KH 8g | EW 57g | F 48g

Preparation time: 40 min + 90 min cooking time
Servings: 8
Difficulty: medium

ingredients

-> Coal distribution: ½ below, ½ on the lid

- 400ml broth
- 6 small onions
- 4 tbsp BBQ rub
- 3 tbsp mustard
- 2 ½ kg pork neck
- 3 tbsp tomato paste
- 2 dried hot peppers
- 2 apples
- 1 shot of sherry
- 1 tbsp hoisin sauce
- 2 tbsp oil

preparation

1.) Put the rub in a large bowl and then turn the meat in it thoroughly and rub the rub. Then let it flow.

2.) Peel and chop the onions. Wash the peppers and cut into strips. Wash the apples as well, remove the core and then cut into slightly thicker slices.

3.) Put the oil in the Dutch Oven and fry the onions until translucent. Add the peppers and apples and fry lightly. Add the tomato paste and mix everything together. Place the meat on the bed of vegetables and pour the broth over everything. Simmer for 90 minutes and then add the sherry. After the cooking time, let the meat rest so that it is easier to pull afterwards.

KH 31g | EW 49g | F 48g

Preparation time: 15 min + 120 min cooking time
Servings: 4
Difficulty: medium

ingredients

-> Coal distribution: 1/3 underneath, 2/3 on the lid

- 600g mixed minced meat
- 100ml broth
- 150g Edam
- 4 slices of pork belly
- 3 large potatoes
- 1 Hokkaido pumpkin
- 2 cloves of garlic
- 1 egg
- 2 chillies
- 1 roll from the day before
- salt and pepper

preparation

1.) Preheat the Dutch Oven. Peel and chop the garlic. Wash the chilies and chop them up too. Wash the pumpkin thoroughly and remove the lid. Remove the pumpkin flesh and set aside.

2.) Mix the minced meat with the roll and egg in a bowl and knead well. Add the cheese and garlic and knead in. Now add the chillies and season everything to taste. Fill the pumpkin with the pumpkin meat you just removed and then sprinkle with cheese.

3.) Line the bottom of the Dutch Oven with the belly slices and then place the pumpkin on top and close the lid.

4.) Peel the potatoes and cut them into slices. Then place around the pumpkin and season to taste. Pour broth over everything and then simmer with the lid closed for about 2 hours.

KH 13g | EW 30g | F 12g

===

Preparation time: 60 min
Servings: 4
Difficulty: medium

ingredients

-> Coal distribution: 2/3 below, 1/3 on the lid

- 500g prawns
- 120ml chicken broth
- 120g pre-cooked rice
- 75g onions
- 50g desiccated coconut
- 2 tbsp olive oil
- 2 teaspoons of cayenne powder
- 2 teaspoons of brown sugar
- 1 green pepper
- 1 egg
- 1 teaspoon thyme
- 1 teaspoon of cinnamon
- salt and pepper

preparation

1.) Preheat the Dutch Oven. Peel and chop the onions. Put the oil in the pot and sauté the onions until translucent. Wash, core and cut the bell peppers. Put the coconut flakes in a bowl. Prepare the shrimp ready to eat.

2.) Whisk the eggs. Turn the shrimp first in the eggs, then in the desiccated coconut. Place the breaded prawns in the Dutch Oven and fry briefly on both sides until they are evenly browned.

3.) Put the onions in the Dutch Oven and also add the peppers. Season the rice with the spices and then place in the center of the pot. Pour the chicken stock over the rice while the vegetables fry on the edge. Close the lid and let everything rest in the pot until the rice is warm.

KH 45g | EW 6g | F 2g

Preparation time: 30 min + 90 min cooking time
Servings: 4
Difficulty: easy

ingredients

-> Coal distribution: 1/3 underneath, 2/3 on the lid
- 500ml vegetable stock
- 150ml white wine
- 5 potatoes
- 2 large zucchinis
- 1 onion
- 2 cloves of garlic
- 1 bell pepper
- 3 jalapenos
- 1 celery
- salt and pepper

preparation

1.) Peel and chop the onion and garlic. Place in the Dutch Oven and simmer until the onion is translucent. Peel the carrots and then dice them. Wash the peppers, remove the core and cut into slices. Then halve these slices again.

2.) Wash off the celery and dice it into small pieces. Then fry in the Dutch oven. Wash the jalapenos and cut into rings. Fry the carrots, bell peppers and jalapenos in the Dutch oven and stir everything thoroughly. Then season to taste.

3.) Now wash the zucchinis thoroughly and then cut them into cubes. Add to the remaining ingredients in the saucepan and let sear for 10 minutes. Then deglaze everything with the broth and add the white wine. Season again if necessary. Simmer for about 1 hour and then serve.

4.) If you want to eat some meat with it, you can fry the bacon cubes .

KH 22g | EW 8g | F 9g

===

Preparation time: 40 min + 30 min cooking time
Servings: 8
Difficulty: easy

ingredients

-> Coal distribution: 1/3 underneath, 2/3 on the lid
- 800ml vegetable stock
- 800ml canned tomatoes
- 400g pasta of your choice
- 200g salsiccia
- 2 tbsp tomato paste
- 2 tbsp olive oil
- 1 zucchini
- 1 carrot
- 1 celery
- 1 clove of garlic
- salt and pepper

preparation

1.) Peel and chop the garlic and onions. Put aside. Wash the zucchini and celery and cut into thin slices. Peel and quarter the carrot.

2.) Preheat the Dutch Oven and add the oil. Sauté the onions and garlic in the oil until the onions are translucent. Then add the carrot and celery and sauté for a few minutes. As soon as both are soft, add the zucchini.

3.) As soon as this is also firm to the bite, push all the vegetables to the side and fry the sausage in the middle. To do this, cut open the casing and press the sausage into the middle in the form of dumplings. As soon as the dumplings are cooked through, add the tomato paste to the saucepan and season with spices as desired. Then deglaze with the stock and the tomatoes.

4.) Put the pasta under the mixture and close the lid. Then simmer for 25 minutes and test in between whether there is enough liquid so that the pasta can become soft.

KH 30g | EW 97g | F 32g

═══════════════════════════════════════

Preparation time: 60 min + 225 min cooking time
Servings: 8
Difficulty: medium

ingredients

-> Coal distribution: 1/3 underneath, 2/3 on the lid

- 3.5kg beef brisket
- 20 prunes
- 3 large red onions
- 4 carrots
- 2 red peppers
- 2 cloves of garlic
- 10 lemons pickled in olive oil
- 1 can of chickpeas
- 6 tomatoes
- 1 bunch of celery
- 1 glass of beef stock
- some olive oil
- Spices at will
- salt and pepper

preparation

1.) Preheat the Dutch Oven and add olive oil. Cut the beef brisket into pieces and fry in them. Peel the onions and garlic, chop them and fry them. Peel the carrots, wash the celery and bell peppers, cut everything into bite-sized pieces and fry with the beef brisket. To taste.

2.) Deglaze everything with the stock. Now add the tomatoes and then close the lid and simmer for 2 ½ hours. Drain the chickpeas through a sieve and dry them briefly with a kitchen towel. After the cooking time, fold in and let simmer for 30 minutes. Season again to taste.

3.) Finally, put the pickled lemons and prunes on top and let the whole boil again for another half an hour until everything is well absorbed.

Soups

KH 11g | EW 40g | F 10g

═══════════════════════════

Preparation time: 15 min + 15 min cooking time
Servings: 8
Difficulty: easy

ingredients
-> Coal distribution: 2/3 under the pot, 1/3 on the lid
- 1kg of chicken breast
- 1kg mushrooms
- 2 large onions
- 3 tbsp rapeseed oil
- 1 bell pepper
- 500ml milk
- 200g peas
- 200g carrots
- 500ml water
- 4 packets of processed cheese
- salt and pepper
- Other spices and chilli, if you like

preparation

1.) First wash the chicken fillet with cold water and dab it with a paper towel. Cut the fillet into small cubes, dry again if necessary.

2.) Put the rapeseed oil in the Dutch Oven and heat it up. Then add the chicken cubes and fry until there is no more liquid. In the meantime, rinse the mushrooms thoroughly and also dice them. Peel and dice the onion. Add both to the meat and simmer until both ingredients get a little color.

3.) Pour water and milk on top and season to taste. Drain the peas, peel and chop the carrots. Add both ingredients to the milk mixture. After 7 minutes, add the processed cheese. Season a little while stirring and garnish as desired. Always make sure that the Dutch Oven does not get too hot and the soup fails.

KH 30g | EW 5g | F 8g

===

Preparation time: 30 min + 60 min cooking time
Servings: 10
Difficulty: easy

ingredients

-> Coal distribution: 2/3 below, 1/3 on the lid

- 2 hokkaido pumpkins
- 3 cloves of garlic
- 200ml cream
- 200g chestnuts
- 1 leek
- 2 onions
- 1 piece of celery
- 3 potatoes
- 1 piece of ginger
- 1 liter of water
- 2 tbsp oil
- Salt and other spices if you like

preparation

1.) Remove the peel and seeds from the pumpkin and cut the pulp into bite-sized pieces. Peel and finely chop the onions and garlic, wash the leek thoroughly and cut into fine rings. Then peel the celery and potatoes and cut them into cubes.

2.) Heat a little oil in the Dutch Oven and heat the garlic and onions in it. Then add the leek, potatoes and celery. After everything has got a nice color, rub off with water. Simmer for about 50 minutes.

3.) Score the chestnuts and put them on the grill for 20 minutes so that the shell can be removed more easily. After the 50 minutes, refine the soup with the cream and season well. Finally, finely puree the soup using a hand blender and add the chestnuts. Let simmer for another 10 minutes.

KH 60g | EW 36g | F 30g

==

Preparation time: 15 min + 35 min cooking time
Servings: 4
Difficulty: easy

ingredients
-> Coal distribution: 2/3 below, 1/3 on the lid
- 375g chorizo
- 2 onions
- 600g sweet potatoes
- 2 cloves of garlic
- 500g potatoes
- 250ml chicken broth
- 250ml milk
- 500g spinach leaves
- Sweet peppers

preparation

1.) Preheat the Dutch Oven. Peel the sausage and cut into small pieces. Thoroughly peel and chop the onions and garlic. Now fry the chorizo with a little oil in the Dutch oven. Then take out and set aside and fry the garlic and onions in the Dutch Oven.

2.) Peel and chop the sweet potatoes and potatoes. Add both to the onions and garlic and season to taste with the paprika.

3.) Deglaze the whole thing with the chicken stock and milk and let the soup simmer for 25 minutes. Then puree the soup. Thaw the spinach at TK. Then wash the spinach thoroughly in a sieve and add to the soup together with the chorizo. Let it stand for 10 minutes.

KH 25g | EW 15g | F 10g

═══════════════════════════════════════

Preparation time: 15 min + 55 min cooking time
Servings: 4
Difficulty: easy

ingredients

-> **Coal distribution: 2/3 below, 1/3 on the lid**
- 450g lentils
- 150g of bacon
- 1.5 liters of vegetable stock
- 1 bunch of soup greens
- 2 tbsp white wine vinegar
- 1 tbsp sugar
- salt and pepper

preparation

1.) First wash the lentils and then leave them to soak overnight. Wash the soup greens thoroughly and then cut into small cubes. Peel the onions from the soup greens and dice them together with the bacon.

2.) Sauté the onions together with the bacon in the Dutch Oven until the onions are translucent. Then add the lentils with the vegetable stock and cook for about 30 minutes.

3.) Put the soup greens in the Dutch Oven and cook for 25 minutes. Finally, add sugar, vinegar, salt and pepper to taste.

Cheese and potato soup

KH 62g | EW 30g | F 95g

===

Preparation time: 15 min + 30 min cooking time
Servings: 4
Difficulty: easy

ingredients
-> Coal distribution: 2/3 below, 1/3 on the lid
- 750g cream double
- 600g corn
- 500g potatoes
- 500ml milk
- 200g Emmentaler
- 50g butter
- 3 onions
- salt and pepper

preparation

1.) Peel the onions thoroughly and dice them. Wash the potatoes, remove the peel and also dice. Put the butter in the Dutch Oven and let it melt. As soon as the butter has melted, sauté the onions in it. To prevent burning, stir regularly.

2.) After 5 minutes add the diced potatoes to the onions. After another 5 minutes, remove the potatoes and flour them. Make sure you use the right dose of flour. Return to the Dutch Oven and add the milk as well.

3.) Finally add the cheese, the double cream and the corn to the soup. Stir everything thoroughly and season the soup to taste. Simmer for 20 minutes until the potatoes are firm to the bite.

KH 15g | EW 5g | F 8g

====================================

Preparation time: 10 min + 20 min cooking time
Servings: 4
Difficulty: easy

ingredients

-> Coal distribution: 2/3 below, 1/3 on the pot
- 1.7kg tomatoes
- 1 onion
- 1 clove of garlic
- 2 tbsp olive oil
- 1 tbsp crème fraîche
- salt and pepper

preparation

1.) Peel the onion and the clove of garlic and then chop them into small pieces. Put the oil in the Dutch Oven and sauté the chopped garlic and onion.

2.) Wash the tomatoes thoroughly with warm water, remove the stalk and cut into small cubes. Then add to the onion and garlic. Season the ingredients to taste and simmer for about 10 minutes.

3.) Add the crème fraîche to the soup and stir everything together. If desired, puree the soup. Simmer for another 10 minutes.

KH 25g | EW 4g | F 16g

═══════════════════════════════════

Preparation time: 15 min + 25 min cooking time
Servings: 4
Difficulty: easy

ingredients

-> Coal distribution: 2/3 below, 1/3 on the lid
- 1200ml vegetable stock
- 750g zucchini
- 300g potatoes
- 200g crème fraîche
- 3 onions
- 1 clove of garlic
- 3 tbsp clarified butter
- salt and pepper

preparation

1.) Peel and dice the onions and garlic. Then sauté with the clarified butter in the Dutch Oven. Wash the zucchinis thoroughly with warm water and remove the ends. Clean the potatoes and then cut them into cubes. The zucchinis too. Add both to the onions and garlic.

2.) After sautéing, deglaze all ingredients with the vegetable stock and simmer for 15 minutes. Then carefully puree with a hand blender.

3.) Now stir in the crème fraîche and mix everything together well and season with salt and pepper if necessary. Let simmer again for 10 minutes.

KH 9g | EW 38g | F 26g

===

Preparation time: 15 min + 300 min cooking time
Servings: 4
Difficulty: easy

ingredients

-> Coal distribution: 2/3 below, 1/3 on the lid

- 1 soup chicken
- 400g carrots
- 1 stick of leek
- 2 ½ liters of water
- 250g pearl barley
- 250g celery
- 2 green onions
- 1 tbsp tomato paste
- 2 tbsp soy sauce
- 2 tbsp oil
- salt and pepper

preparation

1.) Preheat the Dutch Oven, cut up the soup chicken and, as soon as the Dutch Oven has reached a good temperature, add a little oil and let it fry.

2.) Wash the vegetable onions, the leek, the pearl barley and the celery thoroughly with warm water and dice. Wash, peel and slice the carrots as well.

3.) As soon as the meat is through, take it out of the Dutch oven, add the onions and sauté until translucent. Then add the water and stir in the tomato paste.

4.) Add the previously diced vegetables to the pot, season to taste and let simmer for 3 ½ hours. After simmering, remove the meat and detach it from the bone. Put the meat back into the pot and simmer for another 90 minutes.

KH 10g | EW 5g | F 10g

═══════════════════════════════════

Preparation time: 20 min + 35 min cooking time
Servings: 4
Difficulty: easy

ingredients
-> Coal distribution: 2/3 below, 1/3 on the lid

- 1200ml vegetable stock
- 75g rice
- 5 tbsp lemon juice
- 4 egg yolks
- 3 stalks of celery
- 2 tbsp olive oil
- 1 large onion
- 1 large carrot
- salt and pepper

preparation

1.) Thoroughly clean the celery and the carrot, remove the ends and dice. Peel the onion and cut into small cubes. Put the olive oil in the Dutch Oven and sauté the onions until translucent. Then add the celery and the carrot. Deglaze with the vegetable stock and simmer for 10 minutes.

2.) After the 10 minutes, puree thoroughly with a hand blender and add the rice. This has to swell in the soup for 20 minutes.

3.) Open and separate the 3 eggs and then beat the egg yolks in a bowl until frothy. Then add the lemon juice and mix. Season to taste with salt, pepper and 3 tablespoons of broth.

4.) Take the Dutch Oven off the fire and add the mixture you have just made and mix it thoroughly with the other ingredients. Let everything stand for 5 minutes.

Avocado with potato soup

KH 45g | EW 6g | F 20g

Preparation time: 15 min + 25 min cooking time
Servings: 4
Difficulty: easy

ingredients

-> Coal distribution: 2/3 below, 1/3 on the lid
- 1.1 liters of vegetable stock
- 600g potatoes
- 3 tomatoes
- 2 avocados
- 1 onion
- 3 tbsp lemon juice
- 3 tbsp parsley
- 2 tbsp oil
- salt and pepper

preparation

1.) Wash the potatoes and season well. Peel the onion and chop finely. Heat the oil in the Dutch Oven and then sauté the onion in it. As soon as it is translucent, add the potatoes.

2.) Stir in the broth piece by piece and season everything with the parsley, salt and pepper. Let the mixture cook for 20 minutes and then puree.

3.) Wash the tomatoes thoroughly, remove the stalk (possibly also the seeds) and then dice. Wash the avocados as well, remove the stones, remove the pulp from the skin and then dice. It is important that the lemon juice is drizzled on the cubes immediately so that the pulp does not turn brown.

4.) Finally, add the diced tomatoes and avocados to the soup and serve.

Peppery soup

KH 10g | EW 50g | F 62g

═══════════════════════════════════

Preparation time: 15 min + 45 min cooking time
Servings: 8
Difficulty: easy

ingredients
-> Coal distribution: 2/3 below, 1/3 on the lid
- 6 Cabanossi
- 5 spring onions
- 2 large cans of kidney beans
- 2 liters of broth
- 2 teaspoons of mustard
- 1.5kg minced meat
- 1kg of onions
- 1 tube of tomato paste
- 1 can of pickled pepper (green)
- salt and cayenne pepper
- Chili powder
- oil for frying

preparation

1.) Put the oil in the Dutch Oven, crumble in the minced meat and fry it. After the hack is done, take it out of the Dutch oven. Peel the onions and wash the spring onions thoroughly, dice everything and also fry in the Dutch Oven.

2.) As soon as the onions are translucent, add the tomato paste and the previously fried minced meat. Now cut the Cabanossi into pieces about 1 cm thick and add them to the pot. Let everything fry briefly and then pour the broth on top.

3.) Drain the beans in a sieve, add the green pepper and both to the broth. Finally, season with the salt, the cayenne pepper and the chili powder. Mix everything well and let it boil for 20 minutes with the lid closed.

KH 11g | EW 22g | F 37g

===

Preparation time: 15 min + 50 min cooking time
Servings: 8
Difficulty: easy

ingredients
-> Coal distribution: 2/3 below, 1/3 on the lid
- 250g bacon (mixed)
- 750g minced meat
- 5 onions
- 5 liters of broth
- 1kg sauerkraut
- 1 can of tomatoes (peeled)
- 2 tbsp oil
- Sambal Olek and paprika powder
- salt and pepper

preparation

1.) Drain the sauerkraut through a sieve. Put the oil in the Dutch Oven and fry the sauerkraut in it. After a few minutes, add the broth. Put the peeled tomatoes in the pot without draining them and let them boil.

2.) Peel and chop the onions. Dice the bacon. Fry the onions with a little oil in the lid of the Dutch oven until they are translucent. Add the bacon and fry it too.

3.) After roasting, add both to the Dutch oven. Now crumble the mince or shape it into balls, then fry in the lid again. Then add to the sauerkraut.

4.) At the end, add the spices to taste and bring to the boil with the lid closed at medium temperature for 15 minutes.

KH 40g | EW 28g | F 23g

===

Preparation time: 15 min + 55 min cooking time
Servings: 4
Difficulty: easy

ingredients

-> Coal distribution: 2/3 below, 1/3 on the lid

- 500g minced meat
- 500ml vegetable stock
- 4 onions
- 4 potatoes
- 2 peppers
- 2 cups of coffee
- 1 can of tomatoes (chunks)
- 2 tbsp tomato paste
- 1 glass of green beans
- salt and pepper

preparation

1.) Preheat the Dutch Oven. Meanwhile, peel the onions and dice them into small pieces. Peel the potatoes and cut them into cubes. Wash the peppers thoroughly, remove the core and cut into narrow wedges. Wash off the green beans.

2.) Season the minced meat and shape it into small balls. Then put the onions in the Dutch Oven and sauté until they are translucent. Add the meatballs and let them fry. As soon as these are through, add the other previously cut ingredients and the beans to the pan and fry them.

3.) As soon as all the ingredients are seared, add the chunky tomatoes, the vegetable stock and the two cups of coffee. Season with the tomato paste, salt and pepper and then simmer for about 45 minutes.

KH 13g | EW 25g | F 16g

═══════════════════════════════

Preparation time: 15 min + 35 min cooking time
Servings: 4
Difficulty: easy

ingredients

-> Coal distribution: 2/3 below, 1/3 on the lid
- 500ml milk
- 400ml vegetable stock
- 200g parmesan (grated)
- 100g spinach leaves
- 2 onions
- 2 bunches of wild garlic
- 2 tbsp rapeseed oil
- salt and pepper

preparation

1.) Chop some spinach leaves and set aside. Let the remaining leaves boil in salted water for 5-6 minutes and drain them as soon as they are ready and set aside.

2.) Peel and dice the onions thoroughly. Put a little oil in the empty Dutch oven and sauté the onions. After sautéing, add the previously cooked spinach to the Dutch oven and sauté until translucent.

3.) Then fill up with the broth and milk, bring everything to the boil and season to taste. Wash the wild garlic thoroughly and chop it into small pieces. Set aside a little of the chopped wild garlic and parmesan and add the rest to the soup. Puree everything and let it cook together. Serve after about 20 minutes and garnish with the ingredients that have been set aside.

Apple soup with red cabbage

KH 75g | EW 10g | F 2g

═══════════════════════════

Preparation time: 15 min + 60 min cooking time
Servings: 4
Difficulty: easy

ingredients

-> Coal distribution: 2/3 below, 1/3 on the lid

- 500g red cabbage
- 250ml red wine (dry)
- 4 potatoes
- 4 tbsp olive oil
- 3 onions
- 3 oranges
- 3 apples (sour)
- 1 tbsp vegetable stock
- 2 tbsp acacia honey
- 1 tbsp fruit vinegar
- 1 small piece of ginger
- salt and pepper

preparation

1.) Wash off the red cabbage and then cut in half so that the stalk can be removed. Then cut into slices as wide as a finger. Peel and dice the onions. Peel the potatoes and cut into thin slices.

2.) Sauté the onions with the oil in the Dutch Oven and then add the red cabbage and the potatoes and sauté for about 5 minutes. Deglaze the whole thing with the red wine and as soon as it is almost completely boiled down, fill up with the broth. Now season with the honey, the fruit vinegar, salt and pepper and simmer for 30 minutes.

3.) Peel the oranges, squeeze some of them out and add the remaining pieces as whole fillet pieces with the juice to the saucepan. Peel the ginger and apples and cut both into small pieces. Put everything in the pot and let it simmer for about 20 minutes.

Snacks

KH 54g | EW 8g | F 10g

===

Preparation time: 75 min + 40 min baking time
Servings: 8
Difficulty: easy

ingredients

-> Coal distribution: 1/3 underneath, 2/3 on the lid

- 500g flour
- 1 cube of fresh yeast
- 50g soft butter
- 1 egg
- 1 tbsp sugar
- ½ teaspoon salt
- 1 packet of vanilla pudding
- 150g brown sugar
- 3 tbsp cinnamon

preparation

1.) Mix the flour, yeast, butter, egg and vanilla pudding together. Add salt and sugar to taste and cover and let the dough rise for about 1 hour until it has developed to its full size.

2.) After the hour of rest, roll out the dough and divide if necessary. Then brush with liquid margarine so that the filling can stick well. Now mix the brown sugar and cinnamon well together and spread generously over the margarine. Take more or add other spices as needed. Then roll up the dough and cut into pieces of equal size.

3.) Line the Dutch Oven with baking paper and distribute the pieces in it. Ideally so that they don't touch, so that they remain individual pieces. Bake in the Dutch oven for 40 minutes. After the 40 minutes take it out of the Dutch oven and let it cool down. If desired, a topping can be added consisting of 100g powdered sugar, 3 tablespoons of water and a little lemon juice.

KH 58g | EW 14g | F 20g

================================

Preparation time: 60 min + 40 min baking time
Servings: 8
Difficulty: medium

ingredients

-> Coal distribution: 1/3 underneath, 2/3 on the lid

- 500g flour
- 200g milk
- 200g hazelnuts (ground)
- 2 eggs
- 80g butter
- 160g sugar
- 1 cube of yeast
- 1 pinch of salt
- 2 teaspoons of cinnamon

preparation

1.) Mix the flour, milk and 60g sugar together. Meanwhile let the butter melt and then also add to the mixture. Round off the whole thing with the pinch of salt and the egg and add the yeast cube. Knead the whole thing for at least 5 minutes.

2.) After kneading, let it rest until the dough has doubled. Separate an egg for the filling. Mix the egg white with the ground hazelnuts, 100g sugar and the cinnamon well. As soon as the dough has doubled, roll it out generously and evenly spread the filling you have just put together. Then roll it up and cut it lengthways in the middle. After cutting, braid the dough nicely into a braid.

3.) Put the braid in the Dutch Oven and let rise again a little. Mix the egg yolks with a little milk and brush the dough with it. Then close the lid and bake for 40 minutes.

KH 40g | EW 11g | F 25g

=====================================

Preparation time: 35 min
Servings: 4
Difficulty: medium

ingredients

-> Coal distribution: all briquettes below

- 200g almonds
- 90g cane sugar
- 30g vanilla sugar
- 80ml of water
- cinnamon

preparation

1.) Preheat the Dutch Oven well and, as soon as it is at a good temperature, roast the almonds briefly so that the remaining liquid can escape. Then remove the almonds from the Dutch Oven.

2.) Now add the water and mix in the sugar, vanilla sugar and a good portion of cinnamon as you like. Mix everything together thoroughly. As soon as all the ingredients are mixed, add the almonds to the Dutch Oven again and mix them evenly while stirring constantly. Stir until the almonds have completely absorbed the liquid and are nicely caramelized.

3.) The constant stirring prevents the sugar from burning at the bottom of the Dutch Oven. As soon as the almonds are completely caramelized, take them out of the Dutch oven, spread them out on kitchen paper and let them cool.

KH 36g | EW 8g | F 8g

Preparation time: 30 min
Servings: 4
Difficulty: easy

ingredients

-> Coal distribution: all briquettes below

- 250g flour
- 1 bottle of white wine
- 1 tbsp sugar
- 5 hands full of elderflower (freshly bloomed)
- 3 tbsp coconut fat
- some powdered sugar

preparation

1.) Pick the elderflower. These should be large, freshly opened elderflower umbels. Carefully wash them off and dry them with a kitchen towel.

2.) Mix the flour with the sugar in a bowl. Then carefully add the white wine, so that a thin batter is formed. As soon as the smooth dough has formed, dip the individual elderflower bulbs in it.

3.) Put the coconut oil in the Dutch Oven and let it dissolve. Then put in the dipped troughs covered with dough and remove them as soon as they are done and dust with powdered sugar if desired.

KH 52g | EW 5g | F 27g

Preparation time: 25 min
Servings: 4
Difficulty: easy

ingredients

-> Coal distribution: 2/3 below, 1/3 on the lid

- 50ml walnut oil
- 50ml peanut oil
- 250g popcorn corn
- salt
- 50g sugar

preparation

1.) Whether salt or sugar is needed is to be decided according to the respective popcorn preference. Cover the base of the Dutch Oven with equal parts of the oil and heat.

2.) As soon as the oil is hot enough, start with a little popcorn corn. As soon as it pops, the oil is hot enough and all of the popcorn corn can be popped up portion by portion in the hot oil. It is important that the Dutch Oven remains closed and is always shaken a little so that the corn does not burn at the bottom.

3.) As soon as the whole corn is ready, add the salt and the popcorn is ready. If you prefer the sweet version, you can simply caramelize sugar in the oil before the popcorn corn comes into the Dutch oven and only then is the popcorn made. You already have sweet popcorn.

KH 75g | EW 30g | F 34g

Preparation time: 15 min + 20 min baking time
Servings: 4
Difficulty: easy

ingredients

-> Coal distribution: 1/3 underneath, 2/3 on the lid

- 360ml warm water
- 500g flour
- 120g mozzarella (grated)
- 100g parmesan (grated)
- 90g soft butter
- 80g baking soda
- 30g rosemary (fresh)
- 20g of sugar
- 2 liters of water
- 1 packet of dry yeast
- 1 egg
- salt and pepper

preparation

1.) First mix the warm water with the yeast in a bowl until it has dissolved. Then mix the sugar, flour, egg, remaining water, baking soda and a little salt together to form a smooth dough. Season to taste with salt and pepper.

2.) Mix the grated mozzarella with the grated Parmesan in another bowl. Roll out the dough and divide it into 6 equal pieces. Then roll them out again and spread the cheese in the middle. Then shape it into a closed roll and make it long enough to make a pretzel.

3.) Finally, put some baking paper in the Dutch Oven and place the individual pretzels in it and then sprinkle with the washed rosemary. Bake for about 20 minutes and after a quarter of an hour check once whether the pretzels are ready beforehand.

KH 24g | EW 33g | F 50g

═══════════════════════════════

Preparation time: 30 min + 20 min baking time
Servings: 4
Difficulty: easy

ingredients

-> Coal distribution: 1/3 underneath, 2/3 on the lid

- 6 dumplings
- 24 slices of bacon
- 6 slices of raclette cheese
- 6 chilies
- 4 tbsp paprika cream cheese
- 1 handful of cashew nuts
- BBQ sauce

preparation

1.) Brush the Maultaschen with the cream cheese. Chop the cashew nuts and spread over the cream cheese.

2.) Round off the whole thing with a slice of raclette cheese. Wash the chilies thoroughly and either slice them over them, chop them up or use a grinder to pour them over the cheese. Depending on how much heat you can tolerate, take more or less chilli.

3.) Now coat the Maultaschen with 4 slices of the bacon by laying it in a braided pattern. Line the Dutch Oven with parchment paper and add the Maultaschen. Bake for about 20 minutes until the bacon is brown in color. If you like it, you can coat the Maultaschen with BBQ sauce after about 2/3 of the time or simply use it as a dip.

KH 23g | EW 13g | F 14g

===

Preparation time: 20 min + 20 min baking time
Servings: 4
Difficulty: easy

ingredients

-> Coal distribution: 1/3 underneath, 2/3 on the lid

- 250g quark (20% fat)
- 125g cream cheese
- 15g sugar
- 1 vanilla pod
- 1 puff pastry
- 250g raspberries

preparation

1.) Mix the quark with the cream cheese in a bowl and then add the sugar. Mix everything together thoroughly. Scrape out the pulp of the vanilla pod and add it to the quark mixture.

2.) Roll out the puff pastry and spread the cream evenly over it. Put the raspberries in a colander and wash off with lukewarm water. Not with hot water or they will get mushy. Then drain on a kitchen towel and distribute evenly on the cream cheese.

3.) Roll up the dough tightly, but be careful not to tear the dough and then cut it into 5cm thick strips. Place a baking paper in the Dutch Oven and add the snails. When they touch, a wreath is created after baking, which can easily be divided into its individual snails.

4.) Then close the lid and bake for a good 20 minutes. Check in between that they are not already done and if you like it even sweeter, you can mix the icing and pour it over the snails.

KH 45g | EW 17g | F 10g

===

Preparation time: 30 min
Servings: 4
Difficulty: easy

ingredients

-> Coal distribution: all briquettes below

- 750g vegetable fat
- 200g flour
- 200ml milk
- 50ml rum
- 5 large apples
- 4 tbsp sugar
- 3 eggs
- 1 teaspoon of cinnamon
- some salt

preparation

1.) Wash the apples thoroughly and peel them as desired or leave them unpeeled. Poke out the core and then cut into rings about 1 cm thick. Make a mixture from the rum, sugar and cinnamon and let each ring steep in it.

2.) Mix the flour, milk and eggs in a bowl to form a smooth dough and add a little salt. Heat the fat in the Dutch Oven until light bubbles form. With the help of a spoon, gradually slide the apple rings carefully into the fat.

3.) If the lower side has a brown color, turn the rings over once and wait again until a brown color is visible. Then remove the rings and let them drain on a kitchen towel. To make the apple rings taste even better, sprinkle with cinnamon and sugar again.

KH 120g | EW 13g | F 24g

═══════════════════════════════════

Preparation time: 20 min + 25 min baking time
Servings: 4
Difficulty: easy

ingredients
-> Coal distribution: 2/3 below, 1/3 on the lid
- 200g powdered sugar
- 100g milk chocolate
- 250g flour
- 100ml milk
- 90g sugar
- 65g butter
- 1 packet of vanilla sugar
- 2 eggs
- 3 teaspoons of baking powder
- 2 tbsp lemon juice
- some salt

preparation

1.) First make the two toppings. To do this, mix the powdered sugar with a little water and the lemon juice in a bowl and melt the chocolate in another bowl.

2.) In a large bowl, mix the flour, milk, sugar, butter, vanilla sugar, baking powder and eggs together so that a smooth dough is formed. Season the whole thing with salt. Then form even balls out of it and press them flat on the upper side.

3.) Line the Dutch Oven with baking paper and brush it with a little oil. Spread the individual balls on top and let them bake for 25 minutes, checking in between to see whether the balls might not be ready beforehand. As soon as they are ready, take them out of the Dutch Oven and brush with the toppings you made previously.

KH 14g | EW 25g | F 44g

═══════════════════════════════════

Preparation time: 15 min + 20 min baking time
Servings: 4
Difficulty: easy

ingredients
-> Coal distribution: ½ below, ½ on the lid

- 400g Halloumi cheese
- 8 apricots
- 2 tbsp olive oil
- 2 tbsp honey
- 3 stalks of parsley
- 2 tbsp nut spice mixture
- 6 wooden skewers

preparation

1.) The apricots, depending on whether they are fresh or canned, either wash and dice or drain through a sieve. Also cut the cheese into even pieces and then distribute them one after the other, alternately on the skewers.

2.) Mix the olive oil with the honey and coat the finished skewers with it. Then pour the nut mixture over it. If there wasn't a ready-to-buy nut mix, just take your favorite nuts and chop them up to create your own nut mix.

3.) Finally, wash the parsley thoroughly, chop it into small pieces and use it to refine the skewers. Then place on a wire rack in the Dutch Oven and bake for about 20 minutes.

Side dishes

KH 50g | EW 28g | F 6g

Preparation time: 40 min
Servings: 2
Difficulty: easy

ingredients

-> Coal distribution: 2/3 below, 1/3 on the lid

- 500ml buttermilk
- 330g flour
- 2 large onions
- 1 tbsp paprika powder
- Oil for deep-frying
- sea salt and pepper

preparation

1.) Put the buttermilk in a bowl and mix with the paprika powder. Peel the onions thoroughly and cut into even rings. Now soak the onion rings in the buttermilk so that they are well covered and can pull through. Let soak in the buttermilk for 15 minutes and stir occasionally.

2.) Thoroughly mix the flour, salt and pepper in another bowl. Preheat the Dutch Oven.

3.) Pour about 2cm of oil into the Dutch Oven and heat until the temperature measures about 180 degrees. Then take the onion rings out of the buttermilk in portions and turn them in the flour. Then carefully pour into the hot oil and fry the onion rings until they are golden yellow. After coloring, remove from the oil and drain on a kitchen towel.

KH 60g | EW 38g | F 12g

Preparation time: 15 min + 15 min cooking time
Servings: 4
Difficulty: easy

ingredients

-> Coal distribution: 2/3 below, 1/3 on the pot
- 750g fish fillet of your choice
- 3 dry rolls
- 2 onions
- 2 eggs
- breadcrumbs
- oil
- salt and pepper

preparation

1.) First cut the fish fillets very small with a knife. Soak the dry rolls and knead with the chopped fillets.

2.) Peel the onions and cut into cubes. Heat the Dutch Oven with a little oil and fry the onions in it. After about 5 minutes, take it out of the Dutch oven and mix it with the fish fillet roll mixture in a bowl.

3.) Now add the 3 eggs and season everything thoroughly with salt and pepper. Form meatballs from the mass and then turn them in the breadcrumbs.

4.) Put the oil again in the Dutch Oven and gradually fry the meatballs in it. The lid can be closed, but it is not necessary.

KH 22g | EW 6g | F 20g

Preparation time: 30 min + 40 min cooking time
Servings: 8
Difficulty: easy

ingredients

-> Coal distribution: 2/3 below, 1/3 on the lid

- 1.5kg tomatoes
- 750g eggplant
- 750g zucchini
- 400g onions
- 2 yellow peppers
- 2 red peppers
- 1 green pepper
- 6 pickled hot peppers
- 4 cloves of garlic
- 150ml olive oil
- salt and pepper

preparation

1.) Wash the eggplants thoroughly, remove the ends and then cut into cubes. Salt these cubes well and let them steep. In the meantime, wash the tomatoes as well, remove the stalk and seeds, and roughly dice both.

2.) Wash the peppers and zucchinis under warm water, remove the stalk and cut into small cubes. Peel the onions and cut into slices, as well as the pickled peppers. Peel the garlic and dice finely like the previous ingredients.

3.) Rinse the salted aubergine with water and drain. Put some oil in the Dutch Oven and fry the diced garlic and the onion slices in it. Then add all the other ingredients except for the tomatoes and stir well. Under certain circumstances, oil must be topped up at one point or another.

4.) Finally add the tomatoes and season to taste, then simmer for about 40 minutes.

KH 4g | EW 25g | F 37g

Preparation time: 30 min + 45 min cooking time
Servings: 6
Difficulty: easy

ingredients
-> Coal distribution: 1/3 underneath, 2/3 on the lid
- 18 large mushrooms
- 18 slices of ham
- 750g sausage meat
- 250g cheese (grated)
- 200g onions
- 2 tbsp mustard
- 1 egg
- water
- bread flour
- salt and pepper

preparation

1.) Thoroughly wash and clean all mushrooms. Then remove the stems, but do not throw them away. Peel the onions and finely chop them together with the mushroom stems.

2.) Add the bread flour, the egg, the sausage meat and the mustard to the mushroom and onion mixture and knead everything well. Then season with salt and pepper. After seasoning with the mixture, fill the mushrooms and sprinkle all of them with the grated cheese. Now wrap the ham and wrap in aluminum foil.

3.) Place a small grid in the Dutch Oven and place the mushrooms on top. Fill up to the lower edge with water and refill if necessary. Then let the mushrooms cook for 45 minutes with the lid closed.

KH 48g | EW 11g | F 12g

===

Preparation time: 30 min + 80 min baking time
Servings: 4
Difficulty: easy

ingredients

-> Coal distribution: 1/3 underneath, 2/3 on the lid

- 325g flour
- 190ml milk
- 40ml sunflower oil
- 35g garlic butter
- 1 teaspoon of sugar
- 1 cube of yeast
- Fresh herbs of your choice
- salt and pepper

preparation

1.) Put the flour in a bowl and distribute it evenly. Then make a hollow in the middle. Meanwhile, heat the milk and then pour it into the cavity you have just formed. Add the salt and the sugar.

2.) Now crumble in the yeast and distribute the oil on the edges. Knead the ingredients into a dough with your hands until it separates from the wall of the bowl by itself. As soon as all of the dough has been processed into a mass, cover and rest in a warmer place for 20 minutes.

3.) After the resting time, knead the dough again and roll it out using a rolling pin. If necessary, wash the herbs thoroughly and chop them into small pieces. Then spread generously in the middle of the dough together with the herb butter. Finally, seal the dough so that it is shaped like a loaf of bread.

4.) Line the Dutch Oven with baking paper and place the shaped loaf in it. Bake for 80 minutes, but check after about 1 hour whether the bread may not be ready .

KH 50g | EW 20g | F 8g

═══════════════════════════════════

Preparation time: 30 min
Servings: 4
Difficulty: easy

ingredients
-> Coal distribution: all briquettes under the pot
- 400g of cottage cheese
- 200g hearty oat flakes
- 60g corn flakes
- 6 eggs
- 2 onions
- oil
- thyme and parsley
- salt and pepper

preparation

1.) Peel and dice the onions. Wash and chop the thyme and parsley. In a bowl, mix the cottage cheese, oat flakes, corn flakes and eggs together. Mix with the onions and herbs and let rest for an hour.

2.) After the lesson, remove small pieces of the dough with a spoon and shape them into balls. Press the ball flat and then place patty by patty in the Dutch Oven. Meanwhile turn twice. Make sure that the Dutch Oven is not too hot to prevent the patties from burning.

KH 56g | EW 14g | F 30g

Preparation time: 25 min + 45 min cooking time
Servings: 4
Difficulty: easy

ingredients

-> Coal distribution: 1/3 under the pot, 2/3 on the lid

- 1kg of potatoes
- 250g cream
- 1 onion
- 50g butter
- 50g grated cheese
- salt and pepper

preparation

1.) Peel the onion thoroughly and chop it into small pieces. Peel the potatoes and cut into even slices.

2.) Oil the Dutch Oven a little and then cover it with a layer of potato slices. Spread the onions and cream on this first layer and season thoroughly.

3.) Then another layer of the potato slices follows, followed by the cream and onions. Repeat the process until all the ingredients have been used up and there is an even layering. Season again at the end and pour some flakes of butter over the top layer.

4.) Now spread the cheese generously over the top layer and close the Dutch Oven.

5.) The gratin now has to cook in peace for 45-60 minutes, depending on your preference, and is best enjoyed warm afterwards.

KH 11g | EW 5g | F 2g

Preparation time: 35 min
Servings: 4
Difficulty: easy

ingredients

-> Coal distribution: 1/3 underneath, 2/3 on the lid

- 1 zucchini
- 200g mushrooms
- 100g cherry tomatoes
- 1 red pepper
- 1 yellow pepper
- 1 green pepper
- 1 clove of garlic
- 20g feta
- 5 sprigs of thyme
- olive oil
- salt and pepper

preparation

1.) For this recipe, either the lid can be used as a pan or the Dutch Oven can be used as a classic pot. That depends on how fried it should be. First of all, preheat the Dutch Oven.

2.) Wash the zucchini, mushrooms and cherry tomatoes well and dice them. Remove the stalk and seeds from the peppers. Peel the garlic and dice it with the paprika. Put the oil in the Dutch Oven and sauté the garlic.

3.) Then add the peppers, mushrooms and zucchini to the garlic in the Dutch Oven and fry everything. It is important to stir constantly so that nothing burns. As soon as the vegetables are through, add the cherry tomatoes and season to taste. Now put the thyme sprigs in the Dutch oven and let cook for a few minutes.

4.) In the last step, just crumble the feta over the vegetables and let it melt a little.

KH 30g | EW 3g | F 3g

====

Preparation time: 45 min
Servings: 4
Difficulty: easy

ingredients

-> Coal distribution: 1/3 underneath, 2/3 on the lid

- 2 sweet potatoes
- 2 onions
- 1 pumpkin of your choice (recommendation: Hokkaido)
- 4 stalks of thyme
- 3 tbsp olive oil
- salt and pepper

preparation

1.) Clean the pumpkin very thoroughly and cut it in half. Remove the core completely and dice the pumpkin meat with the skin. Peel and dice the sweet potatoes.

2.) Peel the onions and then dice them. Put a little oil in the Dutch Oven and sauté the onions until they are translucent. Wash off the thyme and add it. Then add the diced pumpkin and sweet potatoes one after the other.

3.) Season to taste with salt and pepper and then pour in a little water or, if available, vegetable stock and simmer for about 30 minutes. Then chop it up with a potato masher and season again if necessary.

KH 22g | EW 6g | F 2g

===

Preparation time: 40 min
Servings: 4
Difficulty: easy

ingredients

-> Coal distribution: 1/3 underneath, 2/3 on the lid

- 1kg Brussels sprouts
- 4 tbsp olive oil
- 3 tbsp honey
- 1 tbsp mustard
- salt and pepper

preparation

1.) Preheat the Dutch Oven and then wash the Brussels sprouts thoroughly, if necessary remove the withered leaves and then place them in the preheated Dutch Oven and advise against it.

2.) Now mix the other ingredients together in a bowl. Then season to taste and let it steep briefly. After the Brussels sprouts have been seared in the Dutch Oven, remove them and turn them thoroughly in the marinade. Then return to the Dutch Oven and bake for 20 minutes. You can also bake with cheese if you like.

Pastries & desserts

KH 70g | EW 11g | F 28g

====================

Preparation time: 20 min + 50 min baking time
Servings: 6
Difficulty: medium

ingredients

-> Coal distribution: 2/3 below, 1/3 on the lid

- 1 can of pineapple sliced (260g pure fruit)
- 100g almonds (ground)
- 125g butter
- 125g flour
- 100g wheat semolina
- 200ml coconut milk
- 125g sugar
- 2 teaspoons of baking powder
- 2 eggs
- 100g powdered sugar
- 1 lemon

preparation

1.) First line the Dutch Oven with baking paper. Halve the pineapple slices and line the edge with the semicircles. Cut the remaining pineapple into small pieces and set aside for now. Roast the ground almonds in a pan. Melt the butter and beat it in a bowl with the sugar. Add the two eggs to the mixture one after the other.

2.) Mix the flour, semolina, baking powder and almonds in another bowl. Add the coconut milk and the previously prepared sugar mixture to the mixture and stir well. As soon as it has become a mass, fold in the pineapple pieces.

3.) Then put the dough in the Dutch Oven until a smooth dough is formed. Close the lid and bake for 45 minutes. Let cool after baking. Rinse the lemon and use a grater to rub the lemon zest. Cut the rest of the lemon in the middle and mix the juice of this with the powdered sugar and the zest and pour over the cake as a glaze.

Fruit crumble

KH 85g | EW 7g | F 30g

═══════════════════════════════

Preparation time: 45 min + 35 min baking time
Servings: 8
Difficulty: easy

ingredients

-> Coal distribution: 1/3 underneath, 2/3 on the lid

- 2 pears
- 2 apples
- 250g plums
- 250g apricots
- 2 nectarines
- 250g flour
- 400g sugar
- 100g hazelnuts (ground)
- 200g butter

preparation

1.) Wash all the fruit thoroughly. Remove the seeds and cut everything into mouth-sized pieces. Mix together in a bowl and add 150g sugar. After stirring again, let the mixture stand for at least 30 minutes.

2.) In another bowl, mix the flour, butter, ground hazelnuts and the remaining sugar. Now knead the whole thing with your hands until you have a crumble dough.

3.) Spread the cut fruit in the Dutch Oven and then pour the crumble mixture over it. Now close the lid and let the fruit and crumble mixture cook for about 35 minutes. As soon as a golden brown color has developed, the crumble can be enjoyed.

KH 54g | EW 15g | F 8g

═══════════════════════════════════

Preparation time: 75 min + 40 min baking time
Servings: 8
Difficulty: easy

ingredients

-> Coal distribution: 1/3 underneath, 2/3 on the lid

- 500g wheat flour
- 1 packet of vanilla pudding powder
- 1 package of dry yeast
- 300ml milk
- 1 egg
- 1 tbsp sugar
- 50g butter
- 4 tbsp nut nougat cream
- 2 tbsp cherry jam
- 1 glass of cherries
- salt

preparation

1.) For the dough, mix the flour, vanilla powder, dry yeast, egg and sugar together in a bowl. Melt the butter slightly, heat the milk a little and add both to the other ingredients. Knead everything together thoroughly and then let rise in a warm place for about 1 hour.

2.) Put the Dutch Oven in a warm place. As soon as the dough is ready, roll it out thinly into a rectangle. Gently heat the nut nougat cream and spread it over the top half of the dough, spread the cherries in the middle of the dough and the cherry jam in the lower half. Now roll up the dough widthways. Cut the resulting roll into even pieces.

3.) Grease the Dutch Oven with butter and distribute the pieces with the cut side down. First let the dough rise for 30 minutes. Then close the lid and bake for 40 minutes.

KH 55g | EW 9g | F 35g

Preparation time: 15 min + 50 min baking time
Servings: 8
Difficulty: easy

ingredients

-> Coal distribution: 2/3 below, 1/3 on the lid

- 250g butter
- 250g sugar
- 125ml red wine
- 250g flour
- 100g grated chocolate
- 4 eggs
- 1 packet of vanilla sugar
- 1 tsp cocoa powder
- 1 teaspoon of cinnamon
- 1 packet of baking powder
- 2 tbsp breadcrumbs

preparation

1.) Preheat the Dutch Oven well, brush with butter and sprinkle with breadcrumbs. In a bowl, beat the butter with the sugar until frothy. Then stir in the eggs and add the wine.

2.) Mix the flour with the cinnamon, cocoa powder and baking powder and fold in. Put the finished dough in the Dutch Oven and smooth it out.

3.) Put the lid on the Dutch Oven and let it bake for about 50 minutes. In between, always check whether the dough may have been baked through earlier.

KH 30g | EW 11g | F 5g

====================================

Preparation time: 15 min + 90 min cooking time
Servings: 4
Difficulty: easy

ingredients
-> Coal distribution: 1/3 underneath, 2/3 on the lid
- 1 liter of milk
- 250g rice pudding
- 1 vanilla pod
- 250g mixed fruits
- 3 tbsp sugar
- cinnamon
- salt

preparation

1.) Heat the Dutch Oven and brush it lightly with oil. Pour the milk into the Dutch Oven and add the rice pudding. Heat both together, but don't let them boil. Season the rice pudding with salt.

2.) Carefully divide the vanilla pod and scrape out the vanilla pulp. Add the pulp of the vanilla and the pod to the rice pudding and stir every 5 minutes for about half an hour.

3.) Let the rice pudding sit in the Dutch Oven for an hour. Wash the mixed fruits thoroughly and as soon as the rice pudding is ready pour over them and enjoy together. If desired, the fruits can be placed in the Dutch Oven a few minutes beforehand and warmed up. Finally, the whole thing can be seasoned with cinnamon and sugar.

KH 55g | EW 9g | F 13g

===

Preparation time: 15 min + 50 min baking time
Servings: 6
Difficulty: medium

ingredients

-> Coal distribution: 1/3 underneath, 2/3 on the lid

- 200g flour
- 150ml milk
- 130g sugar
- 100g hazelnuts (chopped)
- 2 teaspoons of baking powder
- 1 packet of vanilla sugar
- 1 organic lemon
- 1 egg
- 500g peaches
- 2 tbsp cane sugar
- 1 teaspoon of cinnamon
- salt

preparation

1.) Mix the flour, milk, sugar, baking powder and vanilla sugar in a bowl. If necessary, chop the hazelnuts and fold into the mixture. Also carefully add the egg to the mixture and mix everything together thoroughly.

2.) Wash the lemon thoroughly under hot water so that the smell comes out. Now rub the zest of the lemon with a grater and stir the zest into the dough. Add a little salt and then transfer the batter to the parchment-lined Dutch oven. Spread until you have a smooth mass.

3.) Drain the peaches and cut them into cubes. Then spread over the dough, sprinkle with cinnamon and the cane sugar. Bake for about 50 minutes and remove from the Dutch oven as soon as it is golden brown.

KH 70g | EW 28g | F 41g

================

Preparation time: 20 min + 40 min baking time
Servings: 6
Difficulty: easy

ingredients

-> Coal distribution: 1/3 underneath, 2/3 on the lid
- 200g butter
- 300g sugar
- 4 eggs
- 125g durum wheat semolina
- 1 organic lemon
- 1 packet of vanilla sugar
- 1kg quark (20% fat)
- 1/2 packet of baking powder
- Some milk

preparation

1.) First melt the butter and then put it in a bowl. Add the sugar and vanilla sugar and mix together.

2.) Now mix the baking powder with the durum wheat semolina and stir into the mixture as well. Wash the lemon thoroughly under hot water until the smell comes out. Then rub the lemon peel with a grater and add the zest to the bowl.

3.) Finally add the quark and some milk and mix everything together until a smooth dough is formed.

4.) Place the dough in the Dutch oven lined with baking paper, close the lid and bake for about 40 minutes. Check in between that the cake has not been baked a little earlier.

Pear cake

KH 57g | EW 6g | F 28g

Preparation time: 20 min + 40 min baking time
Servings: 6
Difficulty: easy

ingredients

-> Coal distribution: 1/3 underneath, 2/3 on the lid

- 750g pears
- 120g butter
- 200g flour
- 80g sugar
- 50g almonds (chopped)
- 40g clarified butter
- 30g of brown sugar
- 2 tbsp pudding powder (vanilla)
- lemon juice
- water
- salt

preparation

1.) Mix the clarified butter, butter, flour and brown sugar in a bowl and knead into a kind of crumbs. Add a pinch of salt. Add about 3 tablespoons of water to the crumbs and mix the whole thing into a smooth dough. Let the dough rest in a cool place for 30 minutes.

2.) Rinse the pears, remove the core and dice. Drizzle with lemon juice immediately after cutting. Mix the pudding powder with the almonds and sugar. Add the mixture to the pears. Line the Dutch Oven with baking paper and roll out 2/3 of the dough in it. Poke a few holes in the dough with a fork. Spread the pear mixture on top and crumble the remaining batter over the pears. Chill the dough in the Dutch Oven.

3.) After about half an hour, the pot can be heated and the cake bake for about 40 minutes. Keep the lid closed as much as possible, but you can check after about half an hour whether the cake is ready earlier.

Chocolate pudding

KH 38g | EW 11g | F 19g

===

Preparation time: 30 min
Servings: 4
Difficulty: easy

ingredients

-> Coal distribution: everything under the Dutch Oven
- 750ml milk
- 150g dark chocolate
- 60g sugar
- 3 tbsp cornstarch
- 2 egg yolks
- 1 pack of vanilla sugar

preparation

1.) First, heat 650ml of the milk in the Dutch Oven. Chop the chocolate into small pieces. Mix the rest of the milk with the starch thoroughly. Then add to the boiling milk and bring to the boil. Then remove the Dutch Oven from the embers.

2.) Separate the eggs neatly and stir the yolks into the hot milk. Avoid the egg yolk from setting by constantly stirring it faster with a whisk.

3.) Stir the crushed dark chocolate, vanilla sugar and sugar into the mixture. Mix everything until you have a thick pudding. Let cool down briefly in the Dutch Oven and then serve.

Rhubarb cake with vanilla

KH 75g | EW 16.5g | F 41g

=====

Preparation time: 20 min + 40 min baking time
Servings: 8
Difficulty: easy

ingredients
-> Coal distribution: 1/3 underneath, 2/3 on the lid
- 1500g fresh rhubarb
- 250g flour
- 300g sugar
- 100g butter
- 100g yogurt
- 100g almonds (ground)
- 60g cornstarch
- 7 eggs
- 2 packets of vanilla sugar
- 1.5 teaspoons of baking powder
- 1 tbsp lemon juice
- 1 pack of pudding powder

preparation

1.) Wash the rhubarb thoroughly and cut into small pieces. Prepare the Dutch Oven and let the coals burn through. Mix the flour, 200g sugar, butter, pudding powder, cornstarch, yoghurt and vanilla sugar to a smooth dough.

2.) Separate 4 of 7 from the eggs and put the egg white aside. Stir the egg yolks into the batter. Mix in the baking powder and mix everything together thoroughly. Roll out the dough on baking paper in the Dutch Oven. Spread the rhubarb on top and bake with the lid closed for about 25 minutes.

3.) Beat the 4 egg whites until stiff, meanwhile sprinkle with the sugar and mix well. Mix in the ground almonds and lemon juice and after the 25 minutes baking time, spread over the dough. Bake for 15 minutes.

Crumble cacke

KH 107g | EW 15g | F 30g

═══════════════════════════════

Preparation time: 100 min + 30 min baking time
Servings: 8
Difficulty: easy

ingredients
-> Coal distribution: 1/3 underneath, 2/3 on the lid
- 900g flour
- 350g sugar
- 300ml milk
- 250g butter
- 100g of oil
- 1 cube of yeast
- 1 pinch of salt

preparation

1.) Warm the milk and crumble the yeast into it. Dissolve the yeast in it and then let it rest for 10 minutes in a warm place. Mix 500g flour, 100g sugar and the oil in a bowl. Round off with a pinch of salt. Add the yeast milk to the dough and knead everything into a smooth dough.

2.) Let the smooth dough rest for 1 hour in a warm place. Knead again and let rise for another 10 minutes. Line the Dutch Oven with baking paper and roll out the dough on top. Cover again and let rise for another 20 minutes.

3.) Prepare the streusel in another bowl by heating the butter slightly. Then process into crumbs with the remaining flour and sugar. Brush the dough rolled out in the Dutch Oven with water and pour the crumble over it. Cover and bake for 30 minutes.

Milletcasserole

KH 30g | EW 5g | F 10g

===

Preparation time: 35 min + 20 min baking time
Servings: 8
Difficulty: easy

ingredients

-> Coal distribution: 1/3 underneath, 2/3 on the lid

- 500g cherries
- 500ml almond milk
- 200g millet
- 100g walnuts
- 5 tbsp honey
- 2 teaspoons of cinnamon
- 1 teaspoon coconut oil

preparation

1.) Preheat the Dutch Oven, add the almond milk and bring to the boil. Put the millet in a fine sieve and wash thoroughly with water. Reduce the temperature to half and then let the millet soak for 20 minutes.

2.) Let the coconut oil melt and chop the walnuts. Then put the walnuts in the coconut oil and mix with 1 teaspoon honey. Wash the cherries thoroughly, cut them in half, remove the stem and stone. Then mix into the millet along with the rest of the honey and cinnamon.

3.) Last but not least, spread the chopped walnuts over the top and, with only 2 briquettes left, bake under the Dutch Oven and the rest on the lid for 20 minutes until browning is noticeable.

KH 24g | EW 8g | F 9g

===============================

Preparation time: 15 min + 40 min baking time
Servings: 14
Difficulty: medium

ingredients

-> Coal distribution: 1/3 below, 2/3 on the pot
- 500g kidney beans
- 200ml milk
- 160g whole wheat flour
- 120ml honey
- 100g chocolate chips (made from pure cocoa)
- 80g walnuts
- 6 teaspoons of baking cocoa
- 4 teaspoons of baking powder
- 4 eggs
- 1 teaspoon vanilla sugar

preparation

1.) Put the beans in a sieve and drain them thoroughly, then rinse again with a little water and dab with a kitchen towel. Put aside.

2.) Mix the flour with the baking powder, the vanilla sugar, the eggs, the cocoa and the honey in a bowl. Add the beans and mix everything into a smooth batter. Now chop the walnuts finely, if desired also chop up the chocolate chips and mix both into the dough.

3.) Place baking paper in the Dutch Oven and spread the dough on top. Bake for about 30 minutes with the lid closed. After the 30 minutes check with a stick and, if necessary, bake again for a maximum of 10 minutes.

KH 75g | EW 23g | F 30g

══════════════════════

Preparation time: 15 min + 25 min baking time
Servings: 8
Difficulty: easy

ingredients

-> Coal distribution: 1/3 underneath, 2/3 on the lid

- 750ml milk
- 400g flour
- 240g sugar
- 150g butter
- 150g raisins
- 12 eggs
- 3 tbsp vanilla sugar
- some salt

preparation

1.) First separate the eggs. Prepare two bowls for this. Add 150g sugar to the egg white bowl and then beat until stiff. Add the flour, milk, vanilla sugar and a little salt to the egg yolk and mix everything together thoroughly. As soon as the dough is smooth, carefully fold in the egg whites.

2.) Put the butter in the Dutch Oven and let it melt. As soon as this is completely dissolved, add the batter and distribute the raisins evenly over it. If it is easier for you, you can mix the raisins into the batter beforehand. Then bake for 15 minutes with the lid closed.

3.) After the 15 minutes, divide the dough into 4 equal parts and let it bake for 10 minutes. Then divide it into small pieces, pour the remaining sugar over it and let it caramelize.

Gingerbread-flavored muffins

KH 52g | EW 9g | F 14g

═══════════════════════════════

Preparation time: 45 min + 25 min baking time
Servings: 8
Difficulty: easy

ingredients

-> Coal distribution: ½ underneath, ½ on the lid

- 350g flour
- 150g maple syrup
- 100g butter
- 100g gingerbread (chocolate)
- 100ml milk
- 50g brown sugar
- 50g apple jam
- 2 teaspoons of baking powder
- 2 teaspoons of baked apple spice
- 2 tbsp orange juice
- 2 eggs
- some salt

preparation

1.) Mix the jam, the baked apple spice and the orange juice in a bowl. Cut the gingerbread into small pieces and add them as well. Let everything steep for about 30 minutes.

2.) Melt the butter and then add the sugar, maple syrup, eggs and milk to a bowl and stir. In another bowl, mix the flour, baking powder and some salt together. Now put the butter mixture and the gingerbread mixture in the bowl with the flour and mix thoroughly.

3.) Spread the smooth batter evenly on the muffin tins and then bake for 25 minutes. Test once after 15 minutes to see if the muffins are not ready beforehand. After finishing, you can garnish as you like.

Closing word

We thank you and hope you enjoy cooking the 111 Dutch Oven recipes. Little by little, the trend from the USA is spilling over to us and is increasingly winning the hearts of camping and outdoor fans. Cooking with the Dutch Oven requires experience and the willingness to try something new and do something new - there are no precise instructions and it cannot be cooked to the minute. The Dutch Oven is as wild and untamed as fire and nature itself, so we can make the most of it.

Just have the courage, try many different recipes and don't be afraid - the Dutch Oven forgives many mistakes and almost always results in a delicious dish.